21 THINGS
YOU NEED TO KNOW ABOUT
DIABETES

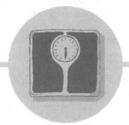

and

WEIGHT-LOSS
SURGERY

Scott A. Cunneen, FACS, FASMBS
and Nancy Sayles Kaneshiro

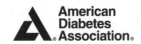
American
Diabetes
Association®

Director, Book Publishing, Abe Ogden; *Managing Editor,* Rebekah Renshaw; *Acquisitions Editor,* Victor Van Beuren; *Project Manager,* Lauren Wilson; *Production Manager and Composition,* Melissa Sprott; *Cover Design,* Jody Billert; *Author Photos,* Dario Griffin; *Illustrator,* Jeff Johnston; *Printer,* Versa Press.

Printed in the United States of America
1 3 5 7 9 10 8 6 4 2

The suggestions and information contained in this publication are generally consistent with the *Standards of Medical Care in Diabetes* and other policies of the American Diabetes Association, but they do not represent the policy or position of the Association or any of its boards or committees. Reasonable steps have been taken to ensure the accuracy of the information presented. However, the American Diabetes Association cannot ensure the safety or efficacy of any product or service described in this publication. Individuals are advised to consult a physician or other appropriate health-care professional before undertaking any diet or exercise program or taking any medication referred to in this publication. Professionals must use and apply their own professional judgment, experience, and training and should not rely solely on the information contained in this publication before prescribing any diet, exercise, or medication. The American Diabetes Association— its officers, directors, employees, volunteers, and members—assumes no responsibility or liability for personal or other injury, loss, or damage that may result from the suggestions or information in this publication.

Erika Gebel-Berg conducted the internal review of this book to ensure that it meets American Diabetes Association guidelines.

∞ The paper in this publication meets the requirements of the ANSI Standard Z39.48-1992 (permanence of paper).

American Diabetes Association titles may be purchased for business or promotional use or for special sales. To purchase more than 50 copies of this book at a discount, or for custom editions of this book with your logo, contact the American Diabetes Association at the address below or at booksales@diabetes.org.

American Diabetes Association
1701 North Beauregard Street
Alexandria, Virginia 22311

DOI: 10.2337/9781580406147

Library of Congress Cataloging-in-Publication Data
Names: Cunneen, Scott A. | Kaneshiro, Nancy Sayles.
Title: 21 things you need to know about diabetes and weight loss surgery / Scott A. Cunneen, MD, FACS, FASMBS and Nancy Sayles Kaneshiro.
Other titles: Twenty one things you need to know about diabetes and weight loss surgery
Description: Alexandria : American Diabetes Association, [2017] | Includes bibliographical references and index.
Identifiers: LCCN 2015018899 | ISBN 9781580406147 (alk. paper)
Subjects: LCSH: Obesity--Surgery. | Weight loss. | Diabetes.
Classification: LCC RD540 .C86 2017 | DDC 617.4/3--dc23
LC record available at https://lccn.loc.gov/2015018899

Table of Contents

Acknowledgments

The authors would like to thank Abraham Ogden, Director of Book Publishing at the American Diabetes Association, who immediately recognized the need for the information in this book; Victor Van Beuren, the American Diabetes Association's Senior Manager of Book Acquisitions, who made the book a reality; and Project Manager Lauren Wilson, for her eagle-eye and thoughtful editing. Thanks also to Dr. Mona Misra, for her cheerful endurance of this process; and to Jenny Arussi, MS, RDN—author of Chapter 20, Food for Thought: A Dietitian's Perspective—for her significant contribution to this project. Finally, the authors would like to acknowledge each other—as doctor and patient, writing partners, and friends.

Dr. Scott Cunneen
and Nancy Sayles Kaneshiro

Preface

If we attempt to address the most important issues facing our country these days, obesity would no doubt make a list of the top five. There are, of course, health problems associated with obesity—diabetes and heart disease, for instance—in addition to the social prejudices against overweight people. So many people think that being overweight is some kind of moral or character weakness.

We know obesity contributes to diabetes—certainly type 2, but many individuals with type 1 diabetes battle the scale as well. Many people with diabetes, not unlike a high percentage in the general population, struggle with losing a significant amount of weight and keeping it off. Obesity is recognized as a potential precursor to diabetes as well as other diseases whose symptoms have severe and often irreversible negative effects on quality and length of life. Weight loss is often vital for people with diabetes or prediabetes.

Most people with diabetes are already familiar with the importance of *lifestyle changes*. For patients who are profoundly overweight, the recommended lifestyle changes—including making appropriate food choices, controlling portion sizes, and getting regular exercise—are difficult, sometimes impossible, to achieve and maintain. Many people with diabetes are, indeed, able to control blood glucose levels with diet, exercise, and medication, but some people struggle.

There have been two relatively recent milestones in the fight against obesity, both of which have had an impact on literally hundreds of thousands of lives in this country. First of all, the American Medical Association has officially recognized obesity as a disease, a move that could induce physicians to pay more attention to the condition and spur more insurance companies to pay for treatments. This heightened focus on obesity is beginning to help improve reimbursement for obesity drugs, weight-loss surgery, and counseling. Secondly, a landmark study by Dr. Walter Pories and associates entitled, "Who Would Have Thought It? An Operation Proves to Be the Most Effective Therapy for Adult-Onset Diabetes Mellitus," has named weight-loss surgery as not only the most effective but also the most durable treatment for diabetes, as it may result in long-term remission for people with diabetes. Scientists are not yet exactly sure why weight-loss surgery is so effective for people with diabetes, but short of an actual cure, long-term remission is the best thing people with diabetes can hope for.

Of course no surgery should be taken lightly. While these operations have become more and more safe in recent years, weight-loss surgery is still surgery, and there are risks associated with it. People considering weight-loss surgery need to determine, with the help of their primary physician and a bariatric surgeon, whether the risk of being severely overweight is greater than the risk of surgery, and whether they are willing to make the commitment necessary for long-term success.

It's important to note that I'm not selling weight-loss surgery in this book. I'm not pushing it, and I'm certainly not trying to represent weight-loss surgical procedures as the be-all-and-end-all solution to our obesity epidemic. Neither is this book a medical textbook. It is my hope, however, that this book will give you information about weight-loss surgery that you might not find elsewhere. I have, in the following 21 chapters, compiled the most often-discussed issues affecting my patients while they are in the decision-making process, while they are getting ready for surgery, and while they're recovering. In this book, I discuss the same subjects that I address with my patients in the exam room or in my office, where they feel comfortable speaking freely.

This book covers the nuts and bolts of the three most popular weight-loss surgery procedures, but it also contains a whole lot of information about *attitude*. "Behavior," "commitment," and "compliance"—these are words you'll see over and over in this book. Surgeons can give you the tool—the anatomical alteration—to succeed, but you need to do the rest of the work. You supply the "guts." Surgeons just move them around a little bit. Weight-loss surgery isn't something surgeons do *to* you or *for* you; it's something they do *with* you. *You* need to make the necessary changes to keep yourself feeling better, looking better, and living healthier in the long term.

This is not an "everything you ever wanted to know about weight-loss surgery" book. It's more of a guide to what your surgeon wants you to know about one of the most important decisions you'll ever make. I hope you will use the information you find here as a springboard for discussion with your own doctor.

Losing weight to reclaim your health requires a huge commitment and a complete change of lifestyle with regard to food. Is weight-loss surgery the easy way out? No. It's a long, arduous process, requiring a lot of hard work and dedication. In the long run, is it worth it? You bet it is!

Scott A. Cunneen, MD, FACS, FASMBS
Director of Metabolic and Bariatric Surgery
Cedars-Sinai Medical Center, Los Angeles

Obesity at Epidemic Proportions

America is not well. We see it in newspapers and magazines, on television, billboards, and bus placards, and, of course, all over the Internet; America is an obese country, and it seems this problem will continue to get worse before it gets better. In terms of the major health risks associated with unchecked obesity, the big-ticket items include diabetes, heart disease, hypertension, elevated lipids (cholesterol), and sleep apnea, all of which can work together to destroy your whole body. However, diabetes and heart disease are the two biggest concerns when it comes to obesity. Even certain cancers have much higher rates in people who are obese than people who are not. If you look closely, you'll see that obesity can cause head-to-toe health problems. The human body is just not built to handle extra weight; it just disrupts and wears everything down.

To add insult to injury, none of us is getting any younger, as I'm reminded every day. As we age, we usually become less active. Our jobs are less active, we don't do as much physical activity, and the aging process itself replaces lean muscle mass with more fat. All of these things conspire, forcing us to eat less just to maintain our weight. Many foods that taste good may be higher in fat and sugar and have more calories than healthier options, so we can't really afford to eat these foods as we grow older.

Fast food can be another obstacle to maintaining a healthy weight; it's plentiful, cheap, and tasty, but it's usually loaded with fat and calories. Many people find it difficult to eat healthy if they're on a tight budget or work long hours and have limited time to plan and prepare meals. It's easier to gain weight if you habitually turn to fast food in a pinch. However, with a little creativity and a lot of motivation, healthy eating *is* possible, even under tight time and budget constraints. The truth is *everyone* has to work hard to keep extra weight off. A genetic predisposition to obesity certainly affects a person's weight, as does how fast the individual burns calories.

"Our society spends *less* on food *per capita* now but the food we purchase contains a lot of calories in a small package."

The reason the obesity epidemic seems worse in this country than anywhere else in the world is because it *is* worse. People are starving in Third World nations. In this country, we don't have a starvation problem to the same extent, but we have the opposite problem. Our society as a whole spends *less* on food *per capita* now than it has in the past, but the food we purchase is mostly calorie-dense food—it contains a lot of calories in a small package, which is a problem. Even with all the health information available to us, we're heavier now than we've ever been, and diabetes and other weight-related diseases have reached epidemic levels. Obesity has actually become America's version of malnutrition.

I am a surgeon who specializes in bariatric surgery, so I'm the guy who performs gastric bypass, adjustable gastric banding, and (the newer) sleeve gastrectomy operations. I'm a weight-loss surgeon, but what I do is really *metabolic* surgery. Sure, my patients show up because they want to lose weight—a lot of weight—but not just because they think they have a shot at being in the *Sports Illustrated* swimsuit edition. They come to me because of their deteriorating health. Most of my patients have diabetes or hypertension, or are at risk for heart attack or stroke. Often their kidneys are failing and/or their hips and knees are shot from carrying so much extra weight. Many have gall bladder problems, back problems, sleep apnea, or any combination of the above obesity-related health problems. Regardless of their age, these people do not feel as well as they should.

Some of my patients come in because they are desperately unhappy. Society in general can be cruel to overweight people. They are stared at, scorned, or thought of as weak and self-indulgent. These people may not interact easily with friends or have a significant other in their lives. Salaries and employment opportunities are often affected by employers' attitudes toward overweight workers, who are sometimes considered to be either lazy or a poor insurance risk that will drive rates up. People who are overweight often feel invisible. Many people who struggle with their weight are unhappy, unhealthy, and uncomfortable in their own skin, and all they want is to be heard and seen for the person they are inside. Some of them don't even know who that person *is* yet! Whatever the reason, whatever the physical or psychological malady my patients bring with them, the common thread is that they want to "fix" the problem. NOW. They've tried everything, they tell me, and now they need help.

Weight-loss surgery *isn't* a quick fix. In fact, it requires a lot of hard work and a lifetime commitment. However, a majority of bariatric-surgery patients significantly improve their health in a very short period of time. Blood glucose levels go down almost immediately after surgery for these people, many of whom have their medications drastically reduced or even eliminated following the procedure, due to a low-calorie post-op diet combined with the hormonal changes created by the surgery itself. Surgery also reduces the high risk of heart attack, stroke, and kidney failure associated with out-of-control diabetes. That can translate into *years* of increased life expectancy for people with diabetes. Losing weight lightens the load on the joints as well, which helps patients get moving and exercise, perhaps for the first time in their lives. Exercise promotes cardiac health and increases lean muscle mass, which, in turn, helps burn calories more efficiently. So it's a win-win all the way around.

Keep in mind that if you choose to explore the surgical route, your surgeon will ask about your level of activity and will want to learn about your particular appetite. The urge to eat is controlled not by the stomach, but by the brain. Long-term weight-loss success is as mental as it is physical. So it's almost as if weight-loss surgeons are trying to accomplish brain surgery by operating on the stomach!

America needs to get well. But getting healthy and *staying* that way isn't easy. I wish I could offer a magic potion or a one-size-fits-all cure that would enable us all to shed weight, keep it off, and lead long, active, and productive lives in great health. Maybe that cure will exist one day, but for today, the solution is just plain hard work. It's meal planning, portion control, motivation, and exercise. It's deciding that the answer to the question, *Do you want fries with that?* is *NO!*

The Skinny on Weight-Loss Surgery

They say *knowledge is power*; no truer words were ever spoken, especially for people who are in the process of making life-changing decisions. Doctors know that the hardest step for many patients to take is the first step through their office door, but we want to make sure our patients get the answers they need. Our work starts by fully informing patients of their surgical options.

A wide spectrum of surgeries exists in the weight-loss arena today, running the gamut from what have been traditionally called *restrictive operations* to procedures that are *malabsorptive*. A restrictive surgery takes your stomach and makes it smaller, so that food sits in a new, golf ball–sized stomach and then empties into your normal stomach to be digested. With a restrictive operation, everything is processed normally after it goes through your stomach, since the doctor doesn't rearrange the intestines. But the actual mechanism creates a complex system of communication within the digestive system—it alters the way your gut communicates with your brain—not just mechanical restriction. On the other extreme, with purely malabsorptive procedures, the patient's mouth is basically connected to the colon. After these surgeries, food bypasses almost the full length of the intestines, so the body doesn't absorb most of the nutrients or the calories in the food that is eaten or experience the same significant hormonal changes seen with the other procedures. Most surgeons don't perform these operations anymore because they're too extreme, and the potential health risks associated with malabsorptive surgeries are great and often outweigh the benefits.

The good news is that today, there are procedures that fall somewhere in the middle of the spectrum. There are "restrictive" operations like the **Roux-en-Y gastric bypass** (named for both a 19th-century surgical pioneer and the configuration this surgery accomplishes) and the **adjustable gastric band**, as well as the very popular **sleeve gastrectomy**. The Roux-en-Y gastric bypass and sleeve gastrecomy procedures combine significant hormonal manipulation with restriction to get the desired results. This means the doctor makes the stomach smaller, so you have to eat differently, slow down, and chew your food well, but the changes to your anatomy also alter how your body processes and reacts to the food. These surgeries create changes in your physiology, resulting in changes to your hunger level and allowing you to be satisfied eating less. The three operations above have proven to have the best risk-to-benefit ratios.

A Bit about the Gastric Bypass

With gastric bypass, the small intestine is cut about 1 1/2–2 feet below the stomach and is attached to a new, small stomach pouch created by the surgeon. The other cut part of the intestine is reattached downstream so that the bile and other digestive juices can flow easily and mix with the food. Food moves from the new stomach pouch directly into a lower part of your small intestine faster than usual. While the bypass and sleeve procedures definitely offer more guaranteed weight loss than the gastric band, they involve a little more early risk because the surgeon is cutting and/or rearranging

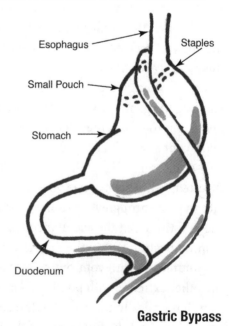

Esophagus

Staples

Small Pouch

Stomach

Duodenum

Gastric Bypass

things. Because the patient's food consumption decreases and the body's absorption of that food is not as efficient, taking vitamins to fill in the nutritional gaps after bypass surgery is non-negotiable for the rest of your life.

A Bit about the Gastric Band

Whereas early restrictive surgeries using bands relied on fixed-sized rings to accomplish their goal, in recent years the restriction has become *adjustable* with the use of the gastric band. One downside of banding is the possibility that you may not lose all the weight you want to, because "cheating" is a bit easier after a banding procedure than after other types of weight-loss surgeries. For example, if you choose to drink primarily high-calorie liquids, a surgeon can never make a band tight enough to stop the liquid; the band has to leave enough room for you to drink water to stay hydrated. So if sodas or ice cream are your weak-

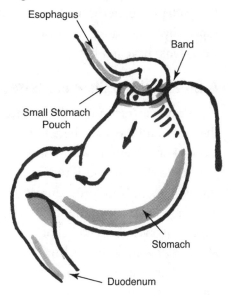

Gastric Band

nesses, you actually might not achieve weight loss even with a correctly adjusted band. If your brain is still hungry after the operation and won't let you voluntarily stop overeating, then a sleeve or bypass is probably a better operation for you. With bypass and sleeve procedures, eating certain types of food may make you sick, so you're "assisted" into making healthy lifestyle changes and losing weight by default, at least initially. The band, on the other hand, allows for less manipulation of your body during the surgery and is, overall, less invasive than other weight-loss procedures. And while you generally get less total weight loss with the band than with bypass or sleeve procedures, you may be able to get enough weight off so that your diabetes is better controlled, and hypertension, sleep apnea, and/or other comorbidities of (or illnesses associated with) being overweight may reverse or significantly improve.

We have to remember, however, that diabetes is a chronic, lifelong disease, and the gastric band is a device that may break and eventually require repair or removal. Therefore, for people with more severe diabetes (and comorbid conditions) who are looking for sustained diabetes control, I strongly suggest gastric bypass and sleeve gastrectomy procedures. These days, I only recommend the gastric band to patients who are unwilling or physically unable to have one of the other procedures. I consider it a better weight-loss option than diet and exercise alone, especially if the patient's previous attempts at attaining and maintaining weight loss have not been successful.

A Bit about the Sleeve Gastrectomy

The sleeve gastrectomy is the surgical option added most recently to the mix—and the one where the amount of achievable weight loss falls somewhere between that of the bypass and band procedures. The sleeve, as it is commonly called, involves the removal of 80–90% of your stomach. The patient winds up with a long tube (the stomach), which is now about the same diameter as the esophagus, that connects the esophagus to his or her pylorus, the opening into the duodenum or small intestine. The patient

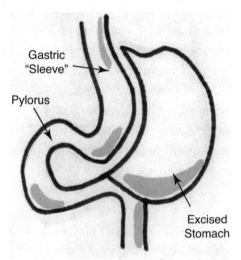

Sleeve Gastrectomy

loses much of the reservoir function of the stomach. The size of the new stomach is about 100–150 cc, or about the size of a small banana or half a can of soda, so it fills up quickly.

Our intestines are not just hollow tubes that absorb and transport things; there are hormones that are released from the intestines that affect hunger, satiety, and how we process foods and sugars. So hunger is regulated by more than just the amount of food we eat. Different kinds of foods trigger those hormones in the intestines. The reduced size of the stomach after a sleeve gastrectomy, coupled with the fact that the portion of the stomach that is removed is one of the places in the GI tract where ghrelin (the hunger hormone) is produced, results in an overall state of altered hormonal balance, allowing you to eat less with less manipulation of the intestines than a gastric bypass requires. The sleeve gastrectomy is now widely used and has become a staple in the bariatric arena. Gastric bypass and sleeve surgeries comprise about 90% of the procedures bariatric surgeons perform, with gastric bands and other procedures accounting for the remaining 10%.

The risk of undergoing a sleeve procedure is about the same as with a bypass. When you cut away the majority of the stomach, you're left with a big, long staple line along the edge of the stomach, and if that doesn't heal well, leaks can occur, creating the potential for infection. And if you happen to have diabetes, you might not heal as quickly as you should. So, while people do like the certainty of weight loss associated with the sleeve gastrectomy, if you have diabetes, are older, and/or are severely overweight, you may be at a higher risk for complications with this kind of surgery.

Conclusion

Most of the weight-loss surgeries performed today combine restrictive techniques and hormonal manipulation to help you reach your weight-loss goals, rather than relying on extreme restriction or malabsorption strategies. All three of these surgeries—Roux-en-Y gastric bypass, gastric banding, and sleeve gastrectomy—are currently done **laparoscopically**, that is, using instruments through very small incisions rather than using the stem-to-stern incisions associated with abdominal surgery years ago. Recovery time for weight-loss surgery is shorter than ever, and the risks of the surgery have been significantly reduced with the popularization of the three minimally invasive procedures discussed above.

But make no mistake about it: all surgeries have risks. All surgeries require careful consideration. And weight-loss procedures in particular require your full attention and commitment. I can't state that strongly enough or often enough. Teaching you all we can about these procedures and making sure you commit fully to the process is how we keep you safe and get you healthy.

Making a
Life-Changing Decision

Most of my patients tell me they've had a weight problem their entire lives. They've tried everything to lose weight, and nothing has given them lasting success. Somehow they've been exposed to the idea of surgery. Some know a little about it, some know a great deal, but for the most part, all of these people want their lives to be improved.

By the time they get to our program, most patients need to lose such a large amount of weight—quite often 100 pounds or more—that it's daunting. Many doctors believe the National Institutes of Health (NIH) guidelines that determined the criteria for weight-loss surgery candidacy, developed in the early 1990s, are in dire need of revision. These surgeries, now routinely done laparoscopically, are much safer today thanks to updated procedures and better equipment. For example, the U.S. Food and Drug Administration (FDA), recognizing the significant health benefit to smaller patients, has now approved the LapBand® for patients with a body mass index (or BMI; an estimated measurement of body fat based on adult height and weight; see BMI Chart on pages 12–13) of 30 kg/m² or above *if* they have comorbidities (conditions associated with obesity). The FDA approved this procedure because it saw that the surgical risk was low and the potential benefit was so high.

BMI Chart

BMI	Normal						Overweight					Obese					
	19	20	21	22	23	24	25	26	27	28	29	30	31	32	33	34	35
Height (inches)	Body weight (pounds)																
58	91	96	100	105	110	115	119	124	129	134	138	143	148	153	158	162	167
59	94	99	104	109	114	119	124	128	133	138	143	148	153	158	163	168	173
60	97	102	107	112	118	123	128	133	138	143	148	153	158	163	168	174	179
61	100	106	111	116	122	127	132	137	143	148	153	158	164	169	174	180	185
62	104	109	115	120	126	131	136	142	147	153	158	164	169	175	180	186	191
63	107	113	118	124	130	135	141	146	152	158	163	169	175	180	186	191	197
64	110	116	122	128	134	140	145	151	157	163	169	174	180	186	192	197	204
65	114	120	126	132	138	144	150	156	162	168	174	180	186	192	198	204	210
66	118	124	130	136	142	148	155	161	167	173	179	186	192	198	204	210	216
67	121	127	134	140	146	153	159	166	172	178	185	191	198	204	211	217	223
68	125	131	138	144	151	158	164	171	177	184	190	197	203	210	216	223	230
69	128	135	142	149	155	162	169	176	182	189	196	203	209	216	223	230	236
70	132	139	146	153	160	167	174	181	188	195	202	209	216	222	229	236	243
71	136	143	150	157	165	172	179	186	193	200	208	215	222	229	236	243	250
72	140	147	154	162	169	177	184	191	199	206	213	221	228	235	242	250	258
73	144	151	159	166	174	182	189	197	204	212	219	227	235	242	250	257	265
74	148	155	163	171	179	186	194	202	210	218	225	233	241	249	256	264	272
75	152	160	168	176	184	192	200	208	216	224	232	240	248	256	264	272	279
76	156	164	172	180	189	197	205	213	221	230	238	246	254	263	271	279	287

National Institutes of Health. Body mass index table. Available from http://www.nhlbi.nih.gov/health/educational/lose_wt/BMI/bmi_tbl.pdf.

However, the American Diabetes Association does not recommend weight-loss surgery for people with a BMI ≤35 kg/m². The association's *Standards of Medical Care in Diabetes* specifies that bariatric surgery can be considered for adults with a *BMI >35 kg/m² and type 2 diabetes,* especially if diabetes or associated comorbidities are difficult to control with lifestyle changes and medication. If your BMI is >35 kg/m² and you already have diabetes, then losing even 50 pounds with weight-loss surgery should treat your diabetes better in the long term than medication alone, meaning your blood glucose would be under better control with weight-loss surgery than if you took medication every day and tried unsuccessfully to lose weight. The relative safety of today's weight-loss surgeries, coupled with the long-term potential benefits of these surgeries, makes the risk assessment equation different than it was more than 20 years ago, when the NIH guidelines were first developed.

All weight-loss surgeries—all of the options to provide weight loss *invasively*—are evolving. The basic concepts are there, but bariatric surgeons are always looking for a better and simpler way to achieve the results. Weight-loss procedures are always going to rely on a combination of several different strategies, including proper eating habits,

				Extreme obesity														
36	37	38	39	40	41	42	43	44	45	46	47	48	49	50	51	52	53	54
172	177	181	186	191	196	201	205	210	215	220	224	229	234	239	244	248	253	258
178	183	188	193	198	203	208	212	217	222	227	232	237	242	247	252	257	262	267
184	189	194	199	204	209	215	220	225	230	235	240	245	250	255	261	266	271	276
190	195	201	206	211	217	222	227	232	238	243	248	254	259	264	269	275	280	285
196	202	207	213	218	224	229	235	240	246	251	256	262	267	273	278	284	289	295
203	208	214	220	225	231	237	242	248	254	259	265	270	278	282	287	293	299	304
209	215	221	227	232	238	244	250	256	262	267	273	279	285	291	296	302	308	314
216	222	228	234	240	246	252	258	264	270	276	282	288	294	300	306	312	318	324
223	229	235	241	247	253	260	266	272	278	284	291	297	303	309	315	322	328	334
230	236	242	249	255	261	268	274	280	287	293	299	306	312	319	325	331	338	344
236	243	249	256	262	269	276	282	289	295	302	308	315	322	328	335	341	348	354
243	250	257	263	270	277	284	291	297	304	311	318	324	331	338	345	351	358	365
250	257	264	271	278	285	292	299	306	313	320	327	334	341	348	355	362	369	376
257	265	272	279	286	293	301	308	315	322	329	338	343	351	358	365	372	379	386
265	272	279	287	294	302	309	316	324	331	338	346	353	361	368	375	383	390	397
272	280	288	295	302	310	318	325	333	340	348	355	363	371	378	386	393	401	408
280	287	295	303	311	319	326	334	342	350	358	365	373	381	389	396	404	412	420
287	295	303	311	319	327	335	343	351	359	367	375	383	391	399	407	415	423	431
295	304	312	320	328	336	344	353	361	369	377	385	394	402	410	418	426	435	443

exercise, and surgery (one that allows for some sort of natural style of eating). There will always be new operations and new devices that become available over time, but the procedures and techniques available to bariatric surgeons today are safe, time-proven options.

Some patients come into my office who are too large for an immediate, low-risk surgery. Unfortunately, it's not uncommon today to see people who are morbidly obese. We've done surgery on patients who are extremely large, some over 600 pounds. The more a patient weighs, the higher the risk of surgical complications, so if we can get some weight off of an extremely overweight person ahead of time, we're going to try to do that. Delaying surgery for 6 months doesn't mean that the patient's journey has been delayed; it just means that when surgery does take place, it will be with less risk. So for people with a body mass index over 50 kg/m^2, surgeons will often try to get them to lose some portion of their excess weight ahead of time. That will make the procedure safer for the patient and easier for the surgeon, who has to deal with the fat surrounding the organs as well as compensate for the limitations of the laparoscopic equipment.

Most people can lose weight with a diet, but many get frustrated because they know the likelihood is that the weight is just going to come right back. But if we put them through a medically supervised weight-loss program, let them know they're going to diet, lose 50 pounds, and then get their surgery and *continue* losing weight, they don't feel as if they've been cheated or put through something without good cause. They know that we're trying to minimize their risk by getting them to lose some weight before going into the operating room.

"Patients are usually very sensible about asking for help. They say, *There's help out there, and I can access it. I should do that.*"

The average age of patients seeking weight-loss surgery is about 40 years. And 80% of these patients are women, usually with a couple of kids, after their fortieth birthday, realizing all of a sudden that they just can't control their weight. They may have taken weight off after their first child, but put on more with the second and just couldn't get it off. Now it seems impossible for them to lose weight. These patients are usually very sensible about asking for help; they don't see it as a failure. They say, *There's help out there, and I can access it. I should do that.* For some men, however, asking for help is considered a sign of weakness. Female patients, in general, seem to be more proactive in terms of improving or maintaining good health. Male patients are usually in more dire straits before they see a bariatric surgeon; they often come into my office only *after* their primary physicians have told them there are serious obesity-related health problems that need to be addressed, such as diabetes or blood pressure issues. For example, a man might come in if his back is out, or he's had a heart attack, or he needs a knee replacement and the doctor will only do it if he loses 50–100 pounds. When they find they can't lose the weight by themselves, these patients will think about asking for help. And some male patients, because obesity runs in their families, have seen what's happened to their fathers or grandfathers, and they see themselves going down that same path. So they come into my office trying to stop it. They know that conventional treatments, like dieting, haven't worked out for them, and they're coming in for what they see as the next step. Or the *only* step.

Occasionally, bariatric surgeons see patients who don't give their health a second thought. They want to have weight-loss surgery just so they can fit into those skinny jeans. Most of the time these are younger patients in their early twenties. However, some of the younger patients we see, even the adolescents, can have obesity-related health problems; a 17-year-old can already have diabetes or be hypertensive. But in general, younger patients don't seem very concerned about their health. They often feel invincible, and it's primarily for cosmetic or social reasons that they come to see a bariatric surgeon at this point in their lives. It's funny, the people who come in strictly for cosmetic reasons are usually relatively thin compared to other patients. Someone may be 20 pounds overweight and want a gastric band just because they've seen a message on a billboard along with a picture of someone who is not that heavy, so they'll think, *I want permanent weight loss. That person is bigger than I am. This should be a piece of cake for me.* Some people mistakenly think of weight-loss surgery as strictly cosmetic rather than something to prevent future health problems or greatly improve existing ones.

No matter what concern causes you to explore weight-loss surgery in the first place, it is important to find a doctor and a program that fit your particular needs. To lose weight safely with a surgical option, you need to make sure, first of all, that you're ready for major surgery. You want to be healthy enough that anything that needs to be optimized prior to undergoing surgery can be optimized. That's why surgeons check not only your heart, lungs, and all of the obvious stuff, but also your head—your mental state, motivations, and commitment—to make sure you understand what you're getting into. Weight-loss surgery requires making permanent changes, *lifelong* changes. If you're not ready or able to make those changes for any reason, then surgery is not right for you *at this time.*

Most people are dealing with a lot of food-related stress in their lives, and if a patient can't cope with this stress before surgery, he or she could have real issues afterward. After surgery, it may become physically difficult to eat. Certain high-fat and high-sugar foods, such as ice cream, may make you uncomfortable and sick if you try to eat them after a gastric bypass; these kinds of foods are no longer your friend. So you may experience a mourning period or even depression following surgery. The weight-loss surgery program you choose should have the ability to identify any potential problems or food-related issues and help you find solutions—whether that means short-term medications, counseling, or support groups. People who struggle after surgery often think to themselves, *Am I the only one experiencing these issues? What's wrong with me?* And a year or so after surgery, new questions can arise: *I've lost the weight but my life still isn't perfect. Am I the only one who's feeling this way?* Counseling and support groups can help patients work through these feelings.

Sometimes after surgery patients forget the problems they faced before the procedure. Let's say, for example, that before surgery a patient was on insulin, could barely get out of bed, and was short of breath after walking a flight of stairs. A year after surgery these problems are infinitely better, but some of the side effects of surgery may make the patient begin to wonder if it was worth it. To help with all of these potential issues, you need a program that's going to be there for you from the beginning and throughout the entire process (we never say "the end," because you're living with this procedure forever). The right program will offer you all the support you need along the way. A program that offers only surgery won't properly prepare you for the changes you're going to have to make and won't properly support you afterwards as you're going through these changes. Do research online and talk to friends to help you gauge what is okay and what is not when shopping for the right program.

I have my own wish list for what I would consider the ideal weight-loss surgery program. For example, it would be great to have a gym that was attached to the program with an exercise physiologist and unlimited access, more patient access to dietitians for personal counseling, and special classes with chef demonstrations (to teach patients a variety of healthy recipes). All of those things would make for a robust program.

Selecting the Right Surgery for You

There are two avenues you can take when looking for a program. As long as your physician is supportive, that is always the best place to start. If you don't consult with your physician, he or she may be upset that you've cut him or her out of the loop. Weight-loss surgery is a major health choice, so you should certainly involve your primary health-care provider in your decision. However, if your physician is not supportive or is of the opinion that there's no benefit to surgery—that you should lose weight with diet and exercise alone, and that if you can't then there's something wrong with you—then you may choose to try to find a new internist, one who will work *with* your weight-loss surgeon in caring for you. My thought is that weight-loss surgeons shouldn't take over your health care entirely. We want to work with the people who have been taking care of your health for a long time. You certainly don't have to give up your other health-care providers to see a weight-loss surgeon!

Many times patients who know someone who has had success with a particular surgery will gravitate toward that procedure, just as patients who know someone who has struggled with a certain procedure will tend to stay away from that surgery. At present, gastric bypass and sleeve gastrectomy procedures comprise about 90% of the weight-loss procedures surgeons perform these days, because many people think, *If I'm going to do something as drastic as have surgery, it had better work. So give me the biggest gun you have to attack this problem.* Some people are embarrassed to come to a weight-loss surgeon. Many patients who come to see us feel like failures because they haven't found success doing what everyone thinks should work for them—an endless cycle of dieting and hard work. They may think, *If I fail with surgery, that makes me an even worse person. I have to lose weight. I can't fail.* These patients may want the "biggest" surgery we can give them, thinking it will maximize their chance of success, but the ultimate choice should be made as a result of collaboration between doctor and patient.

Making the Choice

After walking my patients through all of their surgical options, I try to work with them to see what their expectations, goals, and limitations are. The gastric bypass procedure is, overall, more likely than a sleeve gastrectomy or gastric banding to put diabetes, at least temporarily, in remission, meaning that diabetes medications are no longer needed to maintain normal blood glucose levels (see page 38 in Chapter 6 for more information on diabetes remission). However, the gastric bypass works better for some people than others. For example, people who are younger, haven't had type 2 diabetes for very long, or don't take insulin as a medication are more likely to have a more drastic and durable improvement in their diabetes after gastric bypass surgery.

In terms of total weight loss achieved by patients, there's approximately a 10–15% net difference overall between the gastric bypass, on the high end, and the gastric band, with weight loss from sleeve procedures falling somewhere in between the other procedures [in studies that range from 1 to 10 years following surgery, like the Swedish Obese Subjects (SOS) Study]. It's important to understand that right after surgery, patients get excited to start their new lives. If you look at bypass patients 6 months after surgery, they will often be completely into the new lifestyle, losing weight rapidly, and looking phenomenal. However, if patients don't maintain the healthy habits of their new lifestyle, about 5 years out many start to put some of that weight back on.

> **"Cutting calories and exercising diligently usually give you about a 5–10% reduction of excess body weight. Weight-loss surgery can give you a 40–50% net reduction overall."**

The gastric band, with its varying degrees of restriction and hunger control, offers less predictable results during the first several postsurgical months. We know that patients may not get the same fast results with the band that other weight-loss procedures seem to provide.

Fifteen years after the procedure, most people who have had a bypass have approximately 50% of their excess weight off, whereas during the first year and a half after surgery many are down over 70% of their excess weight. With the band, you usually see a 40–50% reduction of excess weight during the first few years, but that's generally enough of a reduction to significantly improve a patient's health. Because the sleeve gastrectomy is a more recently developed procedure, the long-term results are less defined. To give you some perspective, cutting calories and exercising diligently usually give you about a 5–10% reduction of excess body weight, which in itself can improve health in people with diabetes. Meanwhile, in the long term, weight-loss surgery can give you a 40–50% net reduction overall.

One question I'm frequently asked by patients who are deciding which operation to have is how much pain is involved with each procedure. I assure them that the pain is actually very manageable. However, you have to remember that everyone experiences pain differently. For example, some people are up and ready to start running around almost immediately after surgery—they are a little sore, just as they might feel after doing a lot of crunches—but others experience discomfort for a bit longer. The majority of people take a little pain medication for a couple of days after surgery, and then maybe just at night for a few nights so they can sleep through the pain, but in general, patients just experience soreness similar to what they might feel after a significant abdominal workout. The pain level is about the same even for bypass procedures. The pain originates from the abdominal wall; it's not internal pain.

The patients who generally experience the greatest amount of pain are those who have hiatal hernias repaired at the same time as having a weight-loss procedure done, because the diaphragm is moved around and irritated when the hernia is repaired. This can result in shoulder pain and mid-back pain, though some of the mild shoulder pain people may feel might just be from the inflation of the abdomen during laparoscopy—in other words, it's "gas pain." Fatigue (that can last up to 4–6 weeks), however, is going to be much more significant with the bypass and sleeve procedures than with the gastric band. What we have to remember is that everyone recovers from any surgery at their own pace, so while many people are back to normal within a couple of weeks after a weight-loss procedure, others may become fatigued if they try to do too much too soon.

Many patients are concerned that their age is a factor in deciding which procedure, if any, is best for them. They often ask if I think they're too old for weight-loss surgery. I try to make them understand that the primary reason for weight-loss surgery is to prevent disease and stop the damage caused by diabetes, hypertension, and other comorbidities of obesity. We do check to see that the patients have a decent life expectancy ahead of them, but we're looking for optimum potential health benefits rather than chronological age. I wouldn't perform a weight-loss surgery for someone who had 3 months left to live, but most obese people who have a life expectancy of 5 years or more can benefit from a weight-loss procedure, and now many people are living well into their eighties. I have a healthy 80-year-old patient who has had a gastric band for more than 10 years—you'd never guess she was 80 years old! Even with older people, the benefits of weight-loss surgery can be great. Losing 40–50 pounds can make a huge difference in terms of getting around on arthritic knees or deteriorating hips. So the targets are different for these people.

How old is too old for weight-loss surgery? I think, at the top end, patients need to be able to get through surgery safely, they should not have any disease that's going to shorten their lives in the next year, and, conservatively, they should have a life expectancy of at least 5 years. So that means that 75-year-old women are still candidates if they're healthy. Of course, the younger we can see an adult patient, the better. The earlier we can begin to reverse or arrest the damage caused by obesity, and/or prevent other diseases, the better the long-term outcome.

What You Should Know After Your First Visit

Most people already have a general idea of what weight-loss surgery is before they see a surgeon, so what I want them to know when they leave my office is that there is help for them—even if they believe they've failed in their past attempts to lose weight. I want to make sure they don't feel guilty about taking this route, because it's going to improve their health. But they also need to know that weight-loss surgery is not an easy fix. Your surgeon should make you feel that he or she is there to help and is committed to being there for you in the long term so you don't have to go through this alone. You need to walk out of your first visit to the surgeon's office feeling that your concerns are legitimate, that you're not crazy for seeking surgery to help with your weight, and that improving your health is a worthwhile endeavor. You should never feel guilty about using this option to help you get there.

A Losing Battle: Trying It on Your Own

4

People ask me all the time why Americans, as a population, just can't seem to control our weight. About two-thirds of the people in the U.S. are either overweight or obese. Americans spend more money on weight loss than the national budget of some small countries. We have the benefits of education and the unlimited availability of quality, nutritious food, and we, as a group, shed millions of pounds each year. But most of that weight is regained over time; only 5% of Americans who lose weight succeed in keeping it off. *What is the deal with our weight problem?*

Some people have no clue what it takes to reach and maintain a healthy weight. But most of the people who come into my office have made concerted efforts to get their excess weight off. Many have been dieting their whole lives. They've been on every program available and they've taken weight off, but for a variety of reasons, the excess weight creeps back on. And it's their health that suffers.

Why Does This Happen?

In America today, the majority of people find themselves battling obesity. The consensus out there is that these people are actually struggling with willpower and their own character in the face of gluttony, but in reality people who are battling obesity need to be aware of how the body is designed by nature. Our bodies are designed to react to our environment, and, as health-care professionals have come to learn, they have a sort of "preprogrammed" set point that determines how they're going to handle energy. It was essential to early human survival—in the era when we had to hunt for food—that the body prevent starvation, and all those preventive mechanisms are still in place in the human body, even though food is now plentiful and easily available. While your body functions well at preventing you from starving, unfortunately it can also cause you to gain too much weight. A diet causes your body to believe that you're starving and food is scarce. In response, the bodily mechanisms that prevent starvation can kick in, causing you to fail to lose weight even if you're eating the same amount of calories that worked earlier. Unless they take measures to change their body's physiology, many people are stuck fighting a constant battle against obesity. So, as we understand more about how our bodies function and how they store energy and use energy, we realize that *physiology*, not willpower, is generally governing where weight settles.

What weight-loss surgery does is change your body's physiology to allow you to combat hunger and feel satisfied with less energy stored up in your body (meaning less fat, which is the predominant way the body stores energy). One term that has become a buzzword in today's weight-loss community is the one we just mentioned: *set point*—or the weight at which your body is most comfortable as determined by the amount of energy it stores. When you try to drop the level of the fuel in the tank (your body) lower than its set point, it goes looking for more energy. It makes you hungry. It makes you find food. It makes you think about food all the time. Eventually the body wins, and you end up eating more food and filling the tank back up.

Society frequently portrays overweight or obese people as gluttons—people who don't care enough about themselves or don't have the willpower to give up the pleasure of food. However, the people who are voicing those opinions are generally the ones who don't have a problem with their weight. If people of a normal weight overindulge at Thanksgiving or Christmas and exceed their own set points, it's often pretty easy for them to shed any unwanted pounds because their bodies *want* to be at that lower weight. And the same thing actually applies to people who *are* overweight. They'll often find it relatively easy to take off that extra 10 pounds gained during the holidays, but when they try to get below their regular weight, their bodies fight back and their weight-loss efforts stall. That illustrates the body's adherence to a set point. If the body thinks it's low on energy, it's going to make you hungry. And our current environment, with its easy access to food, especially unhealthy food, is the perfect environment to drive our bodies to create a higher set point, leading to obesity.

Regarding people with diabetes, the hormonal and chemical changes to the body caused by excess body fat result in chronically elevated blood glucose. And one of the consequences of chronically elevated blood glucose levels is that your body needs to produce more total insulin each day to manage your glucose. Unfortunately, insulin is a hormone that can make you hungry and make you gain weight. So, if you're in a state where your insulin level is consistently higher than it would be if you were at a normal weight, you are going to put on more weight. Some of the drugs used to treat diabetes can increase the amout of insulin your body produces, and may result in weight gain.

Childhood Obesity

Childhood obesity is also a big problem in the U.S. and it certainly con-tributes to the obesity epidemic plaguing American adults. It's possible to positively influence a child's attitude toward food, but evidence also sug-gests that it's possible to push the body's set point beyond what it would naturally be, and this can be extremely difficult to reverse later in life. Once the body realizes a higher set point, it doesn't tend to give up that territory, so it's easy for childhood obesity to progress to adult obesity. Fat cells can only hold so much. If they're completely full and about to burst, the body creates more fat cells—more space to store the extra fat being consumed. Once you have these fat cells, they're there; they don't disappear after 6 weeks of dieting. And when they empty out, they send signals to the body, saying: *The reservoirs are low; we need to find ways to restock.* Education is the key to preventing the body from developing this abnormal physiology. If healthy eating habits are taught early enough and are vigilantly upheld, a child can become a normal-weight adult and may avoid diabetes (and other comorbidities of obesity) altogether.

Hunger and Physiology

In the early days of weight-loss surgeries, volume reduction was thought to govern patient success. The prevailing thought among surgeons was, *If you make the stomach smaller, it will be harder to eat and the patient's willpower will take over.* Today, we know that weight-loss surgeries really work well for people when they make patients feel less hungry and satisfied sooner. The volume component is now considered the less important of two factors that contribute to patient success, the other factor being the change to the body's physiology. It's vital for the success of the patient that the body is *happy* at a new lower weight after surgery. If your body isn't happy at its new, postsurgery set point, you're going to gain weight again.

Understanding your motivation for eating is another vital component to success after weight-loss surgery. Even with the new appreciation of the difference between actually no longer being hungry and being stuffed—the difference between physical hunger and *head hunger*—that surgery brings, we know that, when patients get hungry, they may still want to hit a drive-through rather than make healthy food choices. Even if their newfound awareness of hunger drives patients to eat a stalk of celery instead of fast food, that's probably not going to satisfy them. Physical hunger is satisfied by a combination of the *volume* and *texture* of the food ingested, as well as the hormonal effects of the *type* of food ingested. So a high-protein, high-fiber meal will satisfy hunger. But a high-sugar, high-fat meal (like fast food) is tempting because it tastes great and may convince people to eat for reasons beyond hunger.

The human reaction to food is *physiological* with a *psychological* overlay, that is to say, we *like* the taste of food. We may crave tasty food choices (often unhealthy foods) and people are known to eat for reasons other than hunger, but in general, hunger is the primary force driving you to find food. Have you ever been distracted from or unaware of hunger while you're involved in an activity and then, half an hour later, you find yourself thinking about food and considering what you want for your next meal? That, of course, is hunger. The body is very good at regulating hunger, just as it maintains your fluid balance by regulating thirst. When your body needs fluid, you think, *Hey, water sounds like a good idea right now. I'm thirsty!* And you don't just continue drinking until you're filled to capacity; instead you reach a point where your body isn't thirsty anymore, so you stop drinking. Your body works the same way with hunger. It regulates your energy intake by signaling you if you don't eat enough or if you overeat. If you eat in excess of what the body needs, you're eating for pleasure. Obviously, we all eat for pleasure at some point—sometimes to excess—but generally our weight is controlled by physiology.

The physiological changes achieved through weight-loss surgery can help patients with self-control because, after surgery, their hunger is satisfied with less food. However, while weight-loss surgery may help people control the *recreational* eating of inappropriate or unhealthy foods more easily than they could without surgery, these procedures don't solve the problem 100% of the time. Some patients still consume calories even when they aren't hungry. Patients' personal choices, supported by the presurgery counseling/training they receive, come into play when learning what an appropriate meal size is, what the relative calorie counts for different types of foods are, and what foods to stay away from. There are mobile apps and paper journals available to help you keep track of what you eat. Weight-loss operations do not do all the work for you. Long-term results depend on the patient not only learning about portion size, but also making healthy food choices—selecting healthy proteins and complex carbohydrates, and staying away from simple sugars and fats. It's all about retraining your brain.

We may think we're listening to our stomachs, but it's our *brains* that are really driving us to find food. It's physiology and how your brain reacts to your environment that controls your perception of how often you need to find food. This is how your body regulates energy. To demonstrate how this mechanism works, let's say, hypothetically, you had a successful weight-loss procedure. If the physiological change from the procedure were reversed (your body was put back to the way it was before your surgery), you would eventually regain weight. Even if you used all the same skills (portion control, choosing healthy foods, etc.) that allowed you to lose weight and maintain that loss after your surgery, you would still find yourself gradually eating more and gaining weight over time until you were back up to where you started. So it's not just willpower that is responsible for weight loss, though willpower surely does play a role. After surgery, unless the amount of calories that your body expects is delivered each day, your brain is going to tell you

you're hungry. Often, instead of embracing the realization that they don't need as much energy after surgery, patients use visual cues rather than real hunger to gauge how much they eat. For example, you may think, *I have to eat three full plates of food a day* or, in some cases, *I can afford a treat—I've earned it and I deserve it.* Eventually, without daily vigilance, you may break down and start snacking more often and increasing your portion sizes to satisfy yourself

"When you go on a diet, your body is going to turn down the 'thermostat.' You'll need fewer calories to maintain your weight."

emotionally. This indicates that you're confusing hunger with desire. Self-monitoring is essential to successful weight loss; you need to keep track not only of the number of calories consumed but also the composition (and types) of food you eat. Your willpower will be more effective if you are actually aware of what's going into your mouth.

When you strictly adhere to any diet program but your scale refuses to budge, that means your body thinks it's doing you a favor by hanging on to your energy. It thinks the reserve is going to allow you to survive when food is scarce. That mechanism was very beneficial for people during times when food wasn't readily available in large quantities. When your body thinks it's starving—when your weight has changed from what your body thinks its set point should be—it puts the brakes on and refuses to waste as much energy. When you go on a diet and reduce the amount of calories you take in, your body is going to turn down the "thermostat" (use less energy), which means you'll need fewer calories to maintain your weight. While you have to feed your body, you can't feed it excess calories and then expect it to lose weight. If your body reduces its energy use by 25%, for example, then you have to reduce your calories by 25% to maintain your weight if your exercise and activity levels remain constant.

Then you have to add age to the mix. Just because you've aged a year or two since your surgery doesn't necessarily mean that you're going to burn fewer calories. But as you grow older, if you have less lean body mass, less muscle, and more fat, it takes fewer calories to maintain your body. So if you were a 200-pound athlete in high school but now, years later, you're still 200 pounds, you have to remember that because there's more fat than muscle on your body, you need fewer calories to maintain that weight. Plus, as we age we don't move as much as we once did; even if you're only burning a few hundred fewer calories now than you were when you were more active, that's a few hundred calories you shouldn't eat if you want to stay at your present weight. If you're eating 1,500 calories a day, for example, and you have to eliminate 300 of those calories, that's a significant amount of food you're cutting from your diet to maintain your current weight. So it's not necessarily age that is a factor in maintaining weight, it's the fact that older people tend to be less active and often have less muscle mass, so they use less energy.

Do these common obstacles to weight loss make us a nation of failures? No. One of the reasons we have an awareness of the obesity problem in this country is that the average person is now battling obesity. And when the average person no longer wants to say, *It's all my fault,* then we start trying to find scientific reasons why things are happening. That's where we are today. However, there's still a general lack of awareness surrounding the complexities of weight loss. And the issue is not just that many people lack the mental or emotional strength to lose weight; as I've said, everyone who comes into my office has tried to diet. They have spent a lot of money and a lot of effort trying to lose weight, but they're unknowingly fighting against their own bodies, and the body is programmed to win. The body is designed to survive, and diets send it into survival mode. There are strategies that can help people achieve weight loss despite these obstacles, but most people need something much more radical than just willpower to be successful.

And for *some* of these people, weight-loss surgery is the answer.

Looking Inside: Psychology and Weight-Loss Surgery

I've often said that although weight-loss surgeons operate on a patient's stomach, what we're really doing is *brain surgery*. We combat the physiological mechanisms in the brain that compel our patients to eat, and we rearrange the "plumbing" so that they ultimately eat less and are comfortable doing so. Less tangible, however, are the psychological factors that have contributed to patients' unchecked obesity, the problem that brought them into our office in the first place. If we, as weight-loss professionals, fail to delve into these psychological factors—if we don't make a concerted effort to help people deal with, reverse, and eradicate these factors—they will have less success in accomplishing and maintaining their weight-loss goals, no matter what we are able to do for them in the operating room.

One important component of what we do to prepare people for surgery is to complete a psychological assessment. A psychological assessment serves a few purposes. First of all, it gives us insight into whether or not we think the patient has the ability to comply with the lifestyle changes necessary for post-op safety and success. We need to know which patients comprehend what we're doing, why we're doing it, what it takes to achieve and maintain weight loss, and how to avoid hurting themselves in the process.

As you read in Chapter 2, all weight-loss operations require patients to change their lifestyle in several different ways after surgery. You have to make the choice every day to eat healthy foods and stay away from foods that supply empty calories rather than the necessary vitamins, minerals, and nutrients. The mechanics of how you eat also need to change; you

> **"We weight-loss surgeons also encounter people who *yes* us to death. They'll tell us what we want to hear."**

need to chew your food well and eat slowly, or you're going to be in pain. There are people who say, *I don't think that I can follow that rule 100% of the time,* or *I don't think I'm willing to make those changes in order to lose weight.* We explain that these changes are non-negotiable. They're what your body is going to need from you 100% of the time so you don't put yourself at risk.

There are some people who are not willing to make the lifestyle changes necessary for a successful weight-loss procedure, not because they think it will be too difficult for them to make changes, but because they think, *If I'm going to go through something as drastic as surgery, it's going to do all the work for me.* Some people don't want to pay attention to what they eat; they don't want to think about whether a food has a lot of calories or whether it's nutritious or not. They just eat whatever they want. People who take this attitude aren't ready for weight-loss surgery yet. It's important for every patient to understand that, in addition to the surgery, paying close attention to what and how you eat is essential to your success.

We weight-loss surgeons also encounter a fair number of people who *yes* us to death. They'll tell us what we want to hear, which is problematic because it's difficult to tell whether or not these people are actually going to make the lifestyle changes necessary for success. Luckily, most people, when they think about the surgery and the fact that it may affect their lives in a very serious way, tend to tell the truth, especially when they're put on the spot. In response to questions from their surgeon, many people will say things like, *I think I can do this, but I really don't want to.* Or *I'm not planning on giving up potato chips and soft drinks. I read online that a lot of people still drink soft drinks after weight-loss surgery, so I'm going to follow their direction instead of listening to what you're tell-ing me. They got away with it, so I should be able to get away with it, too.* We do the psychological assessment before surgery so that we can weed out these people and get them more education and/or therapy before approving them for surgery—if, indeed, we can ever approve them at all. We perform these assessments because we know that the long-term success of weight-loss surgery depends on changing addictive or poor eating behaviors. It's important to address these behaviors *before* surgery because it's very difficult to do afterward.

A lot of people have learned to consume food as a recreational activ-ity or for emotional support. It's important to understand your personal relationship with food so that your surgeon can tailor your weight-loss program to emphasize your particular needs. If, for example, you're a person who is depressed and treats food as one of your few friends, you're going to need more psychological support, because weight-loss surgery will drastically change the relationship you've been developing with food over the course of your entire life. Weight-loss surgeons rec-ognize that change is very uncomfortable for a lot of people, so we want to make sure that support is there for you, starting from the time of our initial assessment. In addition, there are support groups—available to most people after surgery—which some people find meet their personal needs. There are also people who prefer to learn anonymously and inde-pendently; online resources and support groups can provide that kind of support for these people. If a patient needs ongoing, intensive psycho-therapy, that doesn't mean that he or she can't have weight-loss surgery, but the therapy should be started before surgery and maintained after surgery for as long as necessary.

Weight-loss surgery can be very disruptive to the way patients live their lives. These procedures force people to focus on changing some-thing that they're very comfortable with: their eating habits. After sur-gery you simply *have to eat differently*. There are people who are addicted to food or are compulsive eaters. Those are the people who need extra help after surgery. If food was their best friend before surgery, then their weight-loss team has to find them a new best friend. That may mean getting them hooked up with social outlets that aren't support groups per se, like hiking groups, dance groups, quilting groups, church groups, or whatever positive outlet they find enjoyable. These people may need help finding exciting places to go or things to do to fill the void that they used food to fill before their procedure.

A lot of people who are extremely overweight are socially ostracized, and getting these individuals re-engaged into a network or a group before surgery is an important part of the process, because they may not have the skills to do it themselves. Introducing patients to positive social and emotional outlets and helping them pursue these outlets is essential to long-term weight-loss success. When people are addicted to food, it becomes a crutch that they turn to in emotional situations, whether they feel sad, happy, lonely, or stressed. Without alternatives to food, people with food addictions may feel abandoned, depressed, or anxious after surgery, when excess food is no longer an option. Also, after surgery, food might not give these people the same satisfaction it did before; taste changes are common after weight-loss procedures, so certain foods—while still enjoyable—may no longer ring the same bells they did before surgery. This is all the more reason to provide weight-loss-surgery patients with viable alternatives to food. Weight-loss surgeons need to find out where people with social and/or food addiction issues are psychologically in order to provide them with the personalized support they'll need after surgery

There are those lucky folks, of course, who do not have a food addiction and are not always obsessing about their next meal. For these individuals, food is just one of many different outlets that they can turn to when they are stressed or emotional. These people tend to transition relatively easily into a postsurgery lifestyle because food does not completely dominate their lives. People who aren't struggling with food addiction usually do well after surgery despite the strict rules they need to abide by to achieve weight-loss success.

One other consideration for people struggling with food addiction is the potential transfer addiction from food to alcohol after surgery. Transfer addiction occurs when a person looks for another pleasurable outlet to replace the first addiction. After surgery, when patients have to strictly regulate how and what they eat, they may turn to substances such as alcohol (or drugs) for comfort. Drinking is something you can do by yourself (not that you should), and many people feel good when they start drinking, at least initially. (Many drugs have a similar effect.) Alcohol may satisfy a person's need to "feel better" at first, but, as with food, too much can cause health problems. Too much food can lead to a variety of diseases, including obesity. It's much the same thing with alcohol: drinking a little alcohol socially is usually not a problem, but if you start drinking more and more frequently, that can lead to serious problems. Weight-wise, as your inhibitions are lowered by alcohol, your judgment may falter, and you may be tempted to eat more than you should. Alcohol abuse is just as unhealthy as overeating, if not more so. It's important to note that after weight-loss surgery, the body reacts differently to alcohol. While the stomach absorbs some of the alcohol you drink, after surgery alcohol reaches the small intestine more quickly, where it is absorbed much faster than it would be if it stayed in the stomach, as it did before surgery. The amount of alcohol you drink after surgery will have a much greater effect on you than the same amount did before surgery. Not only does the alcohol reach the bloodstream much faster after surgery, but the alcohol concentration in the blood can be much higher, so a person may get much drunker much faster after a bypass or sleeve procedure. This phenomenon of faster alcohol absorption may lead to increased incidence of alcohol abuse in bypass or sleeve patients. Anyone who has had weight-loss surgery needs to keep that in mind and should be extra careful about drinking and getting behind the wheel!

Another potential complication that people considering weight-loss surgery need to be aware of is the possibility that some patients' mental outlook and perceptions won't keep up with their physical transformation as they lose weight after surgery. If people who are less confident than others or have self-esteem issues don't change their mental state or attitude in a positive way as they lose weight, they'll still see themselves as the same person they were before surgery, and they won't be any happier. They may even spiral down further emotionally or mentally, because now they've lost weight but it hasn't fixed all their problems. This is where support groups, online support, individual psychotherapy, and, perhaps, even antidepressant drugs for a short period of time come into play. Support is essential for the health and safety of these individuals, at least until any issues with self-esteem and/or depression are resolved.

Life is very stressful and nobody is happy all of the time, but in some cases weight loss can help unmask the root of a patient's unhappiness.

Maybe it's a codependent spouse or an abusive relationship that the patient endures only because he or she thought, before surgery, *I can't do better.* After surgery, these people may begin to realize that they deserve better and may want to move on. Learning how to cope with these feelings in a healthy manner is extremely important.

"Make sure to find a program that offers the education and support you need, both before and after surgery."

As you can see, there are a number of reasons why weight-loss surgeons need to evaluate the psychological state of potential patients. Weight-loss surgeons can often spot people who are cognitively impaired and cannot follow directions or are going to need extra help. We can administer psychological tests, in addition to the initial psychological assessment, to help identify people who are maladjusted or those who have routine deceptive tendencies and are just telling us what we want to hear. We can also try to engage any family or friends who come in with the patient to see if we're getting an accurate representation of the patient. Weight-loss surgeons look at any history of hospitalization for psychological reasons in our patients' records. Patients who practice recreational drug use and do not agree to stop will not be considered candidates for surgery until or unless they quit. For patients who smoke, we want them off of cigarettes for at least 6 weeks before surgery in order to decrease their chances of developing ulcers after surgery. If we think a patient is not being truthful about quitting smoking, we'll do a nicotine blood level test. For weight-loss-surgery candidates who smoke or ingest marijuana products to manage chronic pain, many doctors may be more lenient than if these people are using marijuana recreationally. However, just as we ask that patients give up alcohol for a year after surgery (see Chapter 9), they should be willing to give up marijuana. People may not always be up-front with us about whether or not they are using these substances, so we can test for them if we need to.

What I'm describing in this chapter—the measures we take to evaluate and support patients—is, of course, all part of a very comprehensive weight-loss program at a major medical center. There are, I believe, places that rush patients through the presurgery process. And while most insurance companies require psychological assessments before weight-loss surgery, which are often done during a 1-hour interview with the patient and include psychological testing, these assessments can be "rubber-stamped" in 15 minutes. While most of the patients at these places are going to do just fine, people who do need help and support may struggle if they don't get the attention they need. In some cases, that could mean that these people have weight-loss surgery before they are ready and so lose the opportunity to make the most of it. In extreme circumstances, patients of shortcut weight-loss programs may end up getting hurt; something as simple as no one telling them the importance of taking vitamins after surgery can have repercussions. Make sure to do your research before choosing a surgical program/medical center; find a program that offers the education and support you need, both before and after surgery.

The bottom line is, if you're considering a certain weight-loss-surgery program and you're thinking, *Gee, they're asking an awful lot of questions*, that's a good thing! You're on the right track! The more your surgeon and his or her team know about you, the more they can help you achieve your weight-loss goals. A comprehensive program can put you on the road to good health.

A Few Myths about Weight-Loss Surgery

We have so much information thrown at us from every conceivable direction and device these days that it's hard to know what to believe anymore. It just so happens that weight-loss surgery is a prime example of this kind of information overload. From TV programs and commercials to billboards and bus placards, information about weight-loss procedures is everywhere—and this information is not always accurate! So here are some common weight-loss-surgery myths to keep in mind while you're investigating these procedures.

TRUE OR FALSE? Weight-loss surgery is a quick fix. *False!* Many people believe that all they have to do is pick a procedure, and their weight-loss surgeons will do the rest. They think that, after a short recovery, they can just stand in front of the mirror and watch the weight fall off. If that were true, everybody would be doing it! These operations are designed for people who have tried and tried to lose weight and maintain that weight loss but have been unable to do so. What a weight-loss surgeon gives you is the mechanism, the *tool,* to help you achieve your goals. Weight loss doesn't happen overnight; it takes great effort and daily vigilance. And for the people who don't believe that weight loss is hard work, it may not happen at all. Weight-loss surgery is a lot of things…but it's certainly not a quick fix.

TRUE OR FALSE? Weight-loss surgery is only a temporary solution. *False!* Weight-loss surgery is a permanent solution if you make it one! Surgeons would never put patients through the risks and rigors of an operation for a solution that only had a limited shelf life. When surgeons "rearrange the plumbing" with a gastric bypass or a sleeve gastrectomy, they're not fooling around. And when they install a device in the body like a gastric band, they have no intention of removing it (without a very good reason). While we only have a couple of decades' worth of data on the longevity of these procedures, even bands are designed to last a lifetime. But a weight-loss procedure will only be effective permanently if *you* permanently maintain the lifestyle changes necessary for success.

TRUE OR FALSE? Weight-loss surgery is a cure for diabetes. Well, that's false, too, but this one needs an explanation. One of the impacts of these procedures affects patients with diabetes in particular. Because of the hormone changes resulting from a gastric bypass, many patients show immediate improvement in glucose levels, sometimes as soon as the day after surgery. Sleeve patients can see similar changes. The slower, more moderate weight loss in gastric band patients might generally take a little longer to impact blood glucose levels, but these patients, too, should see improvement in their A1C. Rather than a cure, however, endocrinologists prefer to term what many patients enjoy after surgery as a (sometimes) lengthy *remission* of their diabetes. Blood glucose levels often return to the normal range following surgery, and while some people with type 2 diabetes who use insulin may not get off insulin completely, their dosages can often be reduced. For some patients on oral medications, those medications may be cut way back or eliminated entirely after weight-loss surgery. The possibility for diabetes remission is definitely a perk of weight-loss procedures. For example, nearly 72% of obese patients with type 2 diabetes go into a remission lasting 2 or more years after surgery. (See Chapter 8 for a thorough discussion of weight-loss surgery and diabetes.)

TRUE OR FALSE? Weight-loss surgeries carry no risk. *False!* All surgeries carry risk—a fact not widely promoted on the television commercials and billboards that hype weight-loss surgery. The death rate from gastric band procedures, for example, is somewhere between 1 in 1,000 and 1 in 2,000, depending on whom you ask, and is usually associated with deep venous thrombosis (DVT) or clots in the legs, pulmonary embolisms (blood clots in the lung), or some sort of underlying heart condition. The people who experience these complications usually come in with serious, preexisting health problems—usually uncontrolled diabetes and/or hypertension with varying degrees of accompanying illness. Someone between the ages 25 and 40 years, in relatively good health—which describes the average patient who is going to be having weight-loss surgery—is at very low risk for having a problem in a reputable facility. While many weight-loss procedures are performed in small outpatient surgical centers, there are good reasons to choose a program that can admit you to the hospital overnight, especially for people who have significant sleep apnea or any other conditions that make them high-risk for anesthesia. While some younger patients are ready to go right after getting a gastric band, most of my patients feel much better after having spent the night in the hospital under close observation.

Bypass and sleeve procedures are about ten times riskier than bands. However, now that we have Accredited Bariatric Centers of Excellence (a designation given to medical facilities that, by meeting or exceeding exceptionally high standards, offer measurable, high-quality patient care) in the surgical field, weight-loss operations are very safe—on a par with having your gall bladder removed—*if* you go to a larger medical center or Center of Excellence. If you choose a small hospital or a surgical center that does very few of these surgeries, the risk for these procedures may go up considerably.

The bottom line is that there are risks inherent in all surgeries. I strongly urge *everyone* who is considering weight-loss surgeries to discuss the risks with their physicians, who will help them weigh the surgical risks against the potential health benefits.

TRUE OR FALSE? Weight-loss surgery is the easy way out. *False!* Achieving weight-loss success with surgery actually requires quite a bit of hard work and dedication. In assessing patients' qualification for surgery, we do our best to determine their level of commitment to the process. The best programs out there offer a team of dedicated professionals to help with psychosocial assessment, nutritional counseling, and post-op support—a team committed to lifelong patient follow-up and collaboration with all the patients' other physicians. If weight-loss surgeons educate patients about the work and commitment involved at the beginning of the process, their patients have the best chance at changing their unhealthy behaviors and making the most of their procedures. It's not enough to change on the outside; without making changes on the inside, patients have little hope for lasting success.

Hopefully, this chapter has debunked a few of the most common myths and misconceptions about weight-loss surgery. Having a clear picture of what to expect before, during, and after surgery should help you evaluate whether or not weight-loss surgery is the right choice for you, and give you an idea of what to look for in a weight-loss program and facility.

The Downside of Weight-Loss Surgery

There are a few things you need to know about the aftermath of weight-loss surgery. Even though we try to educate our patients about some of the unpleasant things they may experience as a result of their operation, we find that people often are so excited about the positive aspects of weight-loss surgery that they may not be listening as closely as they should to the other side of the story. So let's address a few of the negative aspects of postsurgery life.

Dumping Syndrome

There is one infamous word that affects so many people who are trying to lose weight: *hormones*. When patients eat, the very nature of the bypass operation—and to a lesser extent, the sleeve procedure—causes the food to reach the small intestine a lot sooner than it normally would. Liquids dump immediately into the small intestine, and a cascade of hormonal reactions takes place that affects how you feel. One of these hormonal reactions created after a patient consumes simple carbohydrates is a profound physical response called *dumping syndrome*—an experience with symptoms similar to that of a panic attack combined with the body's response to low blood glucose—that generally leaves the patient feeling sick. (Gastric band patients do not experience dumping syndrome.)

The symptoms of dumping are pretty unpleasant. You may feel shaky, have a fast heart rate, and start to feel anxious and headachy. Many patients break out into a cold sweat and then experience cramping and the feeling of things rushing through the intestines. Finally you get diarrhea. There is also a type of dumping called *late dumping*, which is the result of low blood glucose and generally happens 1–5 hours after eating carbohydrates. The more common symptoms of late dumping are fatigue and weakness, but late dumping may also involve any of the symptoms of hypoglycemia, including shakiness, sweating, hunger, rapid or irregular heartbeat, flushing, and dizziness.

In addition to the body reacting to high-sugar foods, symptoms may be triggered by eating dairy products and certain fats or fried foods, alone or in combination with simple sugars. So junk foods—such as cookies, cakes, candies, and ice cream—and processed carbohydrates—such as crackers, low-fiber cereals, white breads, and white rice—may cause uncomfortable symptoms. When a chocolate chip cookie or a starchy snack like a pretzel causes this kind of reaction, you'll think twice before you're tempted to indulge again.

The amount of time after surgery that people are susceptible to dumping differs from patient to patient, but the average is about a year and a half, after which dumping usually begins to occur less and less frequently before finally disappearing altogether (for all practical purposes). This is how it works for many (but not all) patients. You would think that people would celebrate when they no longer experience dumping, but many patients come to think of it as a "tool" that helps them control what they eat, and they actually miss it when it's gone!

Knowing When to Call the Doctor

Generally speaking, most patients recover from weight-loss surgery very quickly. Most people start feeling a little bit better every day after surgery, so severe pain during the first couple of weeks following surgery could indicate that the surgical connections may be breaking and leaking or not healing. When digestive contents leak outside of the intestine into the abdomen, you get the start of an infection. The body's typical responses to infection include a fast heart rate, sweating, fever, pain, and not being able to take a deep breath. These things are unusual immediately after surgery, so if you experience any of these symptoms, you should go see your surgeon. Any sudden-onset shortness of breath or increased pain levels are signs that you should at least call your doctor. Some serious postrecovery complications—such as twisting of the intestines, which can cause a bowel obstruction, or bleeding from an ulcer—may require a visit to the emergency room. Keep in mind that not everything will go down the way it used to. Fresh, untoasted bread may tend to get stuck. Red meat may not be as easy to eat as it once was. Some people have trouble with white meat chicken or turkey, though dark meat goes down more easily. Overall, if you don't chew your food well and take sufficient time between bites, you may unconsciously swallow something too big, and food may get stuck in your new anatomy. This can cause temporary pain or discomfort. In some cases, a patient may even need a procedure to fish it out.

Can Weight-Loss Procedures Be Reversed?

In extreme circumstances, surgeons can actually reverse a gastric bypass, but in general, we won't. The biggest reason a surgeon would reverse a bypass is if the patient had symptoms of dumping (which are the same as the symptoms of severe hypoglycemia) that just could not be prevented. Diet changes and medications help most people with this problem. But if a patient experiences severe symptoms of dumping every time he or she eats a food with any sugar in it, for example, it's just not worth it. If a patient is having very severe symptoms—for example, if you're passing out, or your symptoms are keeping you from holding a job or driving safely—and a low-carb diet and medications don't help, those are reasons for a surgeon to consider reversing a bypass. Of course, a thorough inpatient evaluation would have to be done in order to rule out all other potential causes for these symptoms. If a patient has ulcers that don't heal, then sometimes re-establishing his or her original anatomy might be an option. Very severe complications from an operation might also convince a surgeon to reverse that operation. But a patient just being tired of maintaining careful eating habits is not a valid reason for reversal.

With the sleeve gastrectomy, the new anatomy created by the procedure cannot be reversed and is yours for life. But most of the unpleasant post-op experiences can be avoided or alleviated if the patient adheres to the new behaviors, or the postsurgery *rules* (see Chapter 9), laid out by his or her surgeon. The gastric band, on the other hand, can indeed be removed. However, if the band is removed, then the patient's anatomy is restored to where it was originally. When the restriction of the band is removed, the patient may stop losing weight and/or regain any weight that was already lost. Weight-loss surgeons endeavor to educate patients about these procedures as completely as possible ahead of time so that patients don't put themselves through a surgery that they don't fully understand or aren't ready for.

Sliming

Sliming is something that can occur after surgery if food gets stuck and blocks off the opening to a patient's stomach. Our bodies are constantly making saliva to lubricate things, and when the stomach is blocked, the body responds by providing extra saliva to try to lubricate the piece of food that is stuck. But because of the blockage, that saliva piles up. When the saliva reaches a certain threshold, it can come back on you, causing discharge of the excess saliva through the mouth. The act of discharging the saliva, or "slime," pushes both *downward* on the blockage and back upward toward the mouth. The offending item usually gets pushed down but the slime often comes up, and even when the blockage is gone, the slime may linger. The restriction involved with gastric banding is tighter, in general, than the restriction with a bypass or sleeve procedure, so more people experience sliming with the gastric band than with the other procedures (especially in the morning). But sliming can happen after any weight-loss surgery. Sliming is a little gross, but it serves as a good reminder to chew, chew, chew your food after surgery. Check out Chapter 9 to learn about some of the other postsurgery eating habits you'll need to adhere to. Don't worry! It will all become second nature pretty quickly.

Bone Loss and Gastric Bypass Surgery

Can gastric bypass surgery cause bone loss? It's possible. That's one of the potential criticisms of the bypass procedure. After this surgery, the body doesn't absorb calcium as well as it did before, which is why it is imperative that patients stay on a vitamin and calcium regimen. This is especially important for women to know, because it's primarily women who are at risk for osteoporosis as they age. This operation may increase that risk. A young woman who gets a gastric bypass may run into problems with bone loss leading to fractures when she is older, despite taking supplements. This is a real issue, but it's a trade-off. When you have weight-loss surgery, you may be increasing your risk for some of these late-in-life medical illnesses, but you're also gaining overall better health as you get older. To say it another way: if you have a gastric bypass, there's a chance you may get osteoporosis when you're older, but you might not even live to an old age if you stay morbidly obese.

Weight-loss surgeons encourage patients to protect themselves from potential bone loss by being vigilant with their vitamins and calcium, and we ask them to have bone studies as they age. If the vitamins and calcium supplements aren't adequate for certain patients, there are medications available now that can help mineralize bones. Bone loss following a gastric bypass is caused more by malabsorption of nutrients rather than malnutrition. Strange as it seems, people who are overweight or obese may actually be malnourished. If you get calories without eating the proper nutrients your body needs, that's malnourishment. So with or without surgery, it's not just calories you have to worry about when you're trying to eat right; you should also make sure you get all of the vitamins and nutrients—including fiber, protein, and essential fats—you need to keep you healthy. We try to stress to all patients that *everyone* has to supplement their diet, but despite patients' best efforts, some issues may still arise later on.

Iron Deficiency and Gastric Bypass Surgery

The body also has difficulty absorbing iron after gastric bypass surgery. While very few people actually need to have infusions of iron because of this, bypass patients definitely need to supplement their iron intake. Female patients who have heavy periods are at an especially high risk for an iron deficiency. Be aware that you can cause harm to yourself after a gastric bypass if you choose to ignore the changes your surgeon and health-care team tell you to make. It's important not to be lax with your vitamin intake, especially with calcium and iron.

While the overall risk involved with weight-loss surgery is low, you have to be sensible and remember that you need to maintain your body a little differently than you did before surgery. If you adhere to the post-surgery measures outlined by your weight-loss surgeon, you can minimize your risk for some of the unpleasant complications and side effects of surgery.

Weight-Loss Surgery and Diabetes

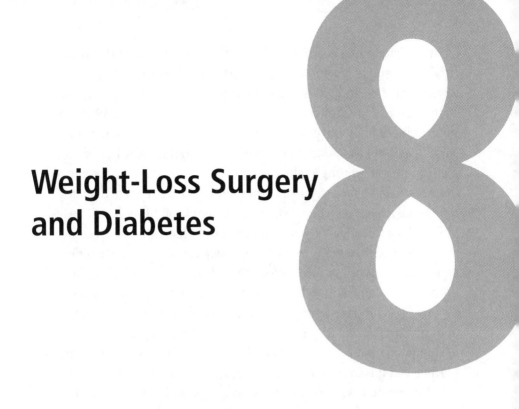

Many people with diabetes have a particularly tough time attaining and maintaining a healthy weight. As we discussed in Chapter 4, if you have diabetes and are on insulin, one of the side effects of the insulin is that it can make you hungry, which can result in weight gain. Many of the oral medications that are used to control blood glucose have a similar effect. It doesn't take very many extra calories to cause the body to maintain (rather than lose) or even gain weight, so many of these diabetes medications can make it more difficult for people with diabetes to lose weight. This is one of the reasons weight-loss surgery is more widely accepted today—by doctors and patients alike—as a treatment for diabetes and other comorbidities of obesity than it was when it was first introduced.

Once the relationship between being overweight and having diabetes was well established and the epidemic of obesity in this country was seen to coincide with the epidemic of diabetes, that's when the benefits, rather than the risks, of weight-loss surgery came into focus. As doctors and patients become more aware that obese people often develop diabetes, suffer heart attacks and strokes, and lose limbs and kidney function, all of a sudden obesity is being treated as a "real" disease, and weight-loss surgery is becoming a legitimate treatment option.

Immediately after surgery, patients may experience diabetes "resolu-tion" as a result of a combination of postsurgery fasting, following a very low-calorie diet, and physiologic changes induced by the operations. Rather than a cure, however, endocrinologists refer to the prolonged improvement in blood glucose control that often follows weight-loss surgery as diabetes *substantial improvement* (significantly less or no medication and improved glucose control) or *remission.* According to the American Diabetes Association, there are three types of diabetes remission: *partial remission,* when the patient is off his or her diabetes medications for at least 1 year and maintains blood glucose levels below the diagnostic thresholds for diabetes; *complete remission,* when the patient is off his or her medications for at least 1 year and maintains normal blood glucose levels; and *prolonged remission,* when a patient experiences complete remission lasting 5 years or more. Many patients in remission feel like they have been "cured," because they are often able to stop taking their medications and their blood glucose levels return to normal. But it is important to note that there is no cure for diabetes.

While we don't know exactly how long a period of remission or improvement will last for individual patients—we don't know if it will last 1 year, 15 years, or a lifetime—we do know that maintaining improved blood glucose levels over an extended period of time will result in less damage to the organs. For many patients, prolonged remis-sion (complete remission lasting 5 years or more) is possible. Prolonged remission gives most patients an even better chance of halting the pro-gression of diabetes-related complications.

Time is of the essence for people with diabetes who are considering weight-loss surgery. And that's why being vigilant about your health—lowering your salt intake, getting your blood pressure under control, and/or taking any necessary medications—is so important. Even though it's not a cure for diabetes, weight-loss surgery can slow down the disease and, in some cases, even prevent its progression. We've all heard of people who have heart attacks with normal cholesterol levels, even if they don't have diabetes or hypertension, so we know that diseases and complications can still happen even if your health improves after sur-gery. But weight-loss surgery can help minimize the negative impact that diabetes can have on your health.

Type 1 vs. Type 2 Diabetes

Having type 1 diabetes means that your pancreas no longer produces insulin. With this type of diabetes, the immune system in your body literally attacks the beta cells (the cells that produce insulin), and your body completely loses the ability to produce insulin. Type 1 diabetes, which most often presents in children and young adults but can occur at any age, results in patients becoming completely dependent on an external source of insulin, either injections or an insulin pump. If you've been diagnosed with type 2 diabetes, on the other hand, the problem is not that your body can't *make* insulin, it's that your body can't use it effectively. Your pancreas still manufactures insulin, just not at a high enough rate to meet the body's needs and control your blood glucose.

In either case, it is crucial to gain control of your blood glucose levels through diet and exercise, oral medication, and/or insulin. Now, weight-loss surgery (or, as it is sometimes called, *metabolic* surgery) has been added to the list of glucose management options for certain obese patients because it has been shown to be a durable and effective "treatment" for diabetes as well as other metabolic conditions.

In people with advanced type 2 diabetes who are on insulin, weight-loss surgery can augment or supplement the *action* of the insulin they're injecting in order to help control their blood glucose. We've found that these surgeries can also greatly improve the body's response to injected insulin, which means that patients can often achieve better blood glucose control using less medication than they did before surgery, though they may not be able to stop taking insulin altogether. If a patient had to take hundreds of units of insulin before surgery, for example, but only needs 20 units after surgery, that indicates that his or her blood glucose levels are more predictable and under better control than they were before—and that's generally when people do better not only with glucose control, but also with avoiding diabetes-related symptoms and complications over the long term. The real problem with diabetes is that if your blood glucose levels are too high on average for too long, it damages your small and large blood vessels, which can lead to long-term damage to your organs.

All people with diabetes need to keep their blood glucose levels under control in order to minimize organ damage and reduce their risk of diabetes complications. People with type 2 diabetes often come to see weight-loss surgeons because they are having difficulty controlling their blood glucose with lifestyle or medication therapy. Surgery may be an appropriate option for some of these people. Some morbidly obese patients with type 1 diabetes are also candidates for surgery, though it's important to remember that all weight-loss-surgery patients with type 1 diabetes will always need to use insulin to control their blood glucose. Being overweight/obese is a major risk factor for long-term diabetes-related damage. By improving the body's reaction to injected insulin, weight-loss surgery can help these people normalize their blood glucose.

Diabetes is a disease that causes the blood vessels in the body to constrict, limiting the amount of oxygen and nutrients that can reach the organs. When the body can't deliver enough oxygen and nutrients to your tissue—whether it's the tissue in the tips of your fingers and toes or in your heart and brain—that tissue starts to die. This is how diabetes complications such as retinopathy and blindness, kidney failure and neuropathy begin.

Weight-loss surgeries change your body's physiology by altering your hormones—which are the signals that allow different parts of your body to communicate with one another—in a way that makes you more sensitive to the insulin that you're administering or producing (if you have type 2 diabetes). These operations change the release pattern of certain hormones from the gut that "talk" to different tissues in your body, such as your brain, liver, intestines, and muscles. These hormones give instructions to the various tissues on how to use insulin more effectively—in essence, they help to normalize a person's physiology. The result for many patients with diabetes who opt for either a gastric bypass or a sleeve gastrectomy is an immediate and prolonged improvement in their blood glucose control. I've had patients with type 1 diabetes who are able to reduce the amount of insulin they take after surgery, and I've had many patients with type 2 diabetes who are able to stop taking their medications entirely.

We all know that exercise is fabulous for everyone's health, including people with diabetes. The more exercise you are able to do, the better the effect on your blood glucose levels. Unfortunately, people with diabetes who are overweight may not be able to take full advantage of the health benefits of sustained exercise and its natural effect of reducing blood glucose levels. A person who weighs 300 pounds, for example, may not be able to accomplish as much in the gym as a person who weighs 200 pounds or less. However, significant weight loss and the change in physiology achieved through weight-loss surgery, particularly with gastric bypass and sleeve gastrectomy procedures, can help. Not only does weight-loss surgery drive blood glucose levels down and help the body use insulin more effectively, it also allows some patients to move and exercise more freely after losing some weight. This is what helps those with type 2 diabetes do so well after weight-loss surgery; exercise becomes safer and easier and, therefore, patients are more likely to exercise on a regular basis.

About 30% of my patients have diabetes, and a good portion of them have started using insulin by the time they come into my office. This chapter has already touched on the fact that people with type 1 diabetes will not be able to stop injecting insulin following weight-loss surgery, but it's important to note that some people with type 2 diabetes may be in a similar situation. Part of the problem with having type 2 diabetes and being overweight with insulin resistance is that your body tries to compensate by producing a lot of insulin, which can overwork the pancreas. One school of thought is that if the pancreas is overworked for too long, it will "burn out" and stop producing insulin. If a person's pancreas stops producing insulin, it's effectively the same as if that person had type 1 diabetes; while that person does not experience the same auto-immune phenomenon you find in people with type 1 diabetes, the results of pancreas burnout and type 1 diabetes are the same. So some people who have type 2 diabetes and who have been on insulin for a long time may never be able to get off insulin entirely, even after having weight-loss surgery. Once the insulin-producing cells in the pancreas are dead, they don't come back. But weight-loss surgery can still do a lot of good for these people by helping them gain better control over their blood glucose.

Gastric bypass is slightly more beneficial when it comes to the treatment of diabetes than the sleeve gastrectomy, but patients with diabetes can still see significant improvement in their blood glucose control with the sleeve. With the gastric band, the hormonal changes caused by surgery are much less substantial, so for patients with diabetes, the improvement in their blood glucose levels is not as dramatic or instantaneous. Two things people with diabetes need to control are their intake of calories and the *types* of food that they eat. Their calorie intake should be consistent and predictable, and because different foods are absorbed by the body at different rates, they should learn to avoid or limit certain types of food. For example, people with diabetes should try to stay away from simple sugars and foods that contain too much fat.

The adjustable gastric band immediately causes a restriction in the stomach that helps patients eat fewer calories and maintain a consistent calorie intake. When a band is appropriately adjusted and working as it was designed to, patients find themselves less hungry and satisfied with smaller portions. One of the benefits of this low and consistent calorie intake is that you often need less insulin or lower doses of oral medication to manage your blood glucose than you did before surgery. A secondary effect of the gastric band is that, as you lose weight, there is less of your body that you have to medicate in order to manage your blood glucose. So while you may not see the same rapid improvement in blood glucose levels with a gastric band as you might with another weight-loss procedure, the band can still result in lower blood glucose levels and the reduction or elimination of diabetes medications.

New recommendations, published in the journal *Diabetes Care*, suggest that weight-loss surgery should become a more routine treatment option for diabetes. Bariatric surgery is recommended for patients whose BMI is at least 40 kg/m^2, regardless of their overall blood glucose levels, and for patients with a BMI of at least 35 kg/m^2 whose diabetes is inadequately controlled despite lifestyle changes and medication. But the new recommendations say that bariatric surgery can also be considered in patients with a BMI as low as 30 kg/m^2 if they have poor diabetes control despite usual care. These new recommendations were endorsed by the American Diabetes Association (though they are not currently official guidelines of the Association), the International Diabetes Federation, and 43 other health groups.

As surgeons, it's our job to "deconstruct" and analyze these procedures so that we can determine which aspects of each surgery offer the most significant contribution in terms of diabetes treatment. It is essential for us to understand how we can maximize the results of these surgeries for people with diabetes. With enough analysis, we hope to be able to determine which patients will respond best to each of these operations.

Post-Op Rules

There are rules that weight-loss surgeons expect patients to follow after surgery, and patients need to stick to these rules for the rest of their lives. They are *lifestyle changes*. These rules vary slightly between the surgical practices and each weight-loss procedure, but they are essentially variations on the same theme. Here are what I consider to be the **Top Ten Post-Op Rules**:

1. *Eat slowly and chew well.* Yes, that's rule number one, and it's a rule that patients need to follow for their entire lifetime. It's a change in habit that must be followed after the surgery is complete. Unfortunately, many people have a habit of not chewing their food well, usually because people tend to eat very quickly when they're on the run and don't pay attention to chewing. All weight-loss procedures (gastric bypass, sleeve gastrectomy, and the gastric band) actually reduce the size of your stomach and, therefore, the volume of your stomach. So if you swallow a big chunk of food after surgery, it can get stuck and cause problems. It will create a plug, just as if you had a clog in the drain under your sink. This will be uncomfortable because your

saliva and other digestive juices are still being manufactured and may back up around the blockage. The body's first response to its new, smaller stomach being overstretched is to create pressure, then pain, and then vomiting. And if you swallow something *really* big, those responses will all happen as one continuous process. So follow this rule!

Chewing well will eventually become second nature; it's a habit that people pick up relatively quickly because the feedback is immediate and consistent. But in the beginning you must be careful to follow this rule, because the body won't negotiate. No one wants to have to jump up from the table to throw up when they're eating with friends. Patients adapt to this rule quickly and most foods can be chewed up effectively, but there are times that you're out with friends or family, and people are talking at you from all directions, when you may swallow without thinking. So I always recommend to patients that if they're going out and find themselves in a situation where they're going to be distracted, they should opt for softer foods. Soups seem to work best.

All weight-loss surgeries will eventually force you to change the way you eat. A good rule of thumb is that a meal should consist of a salad plate of food with a deck-of-cards-size portion of protein (beef, pork, lamb, chicken, or fish), and you should plan 30 minutes to eat it. You should end up chewing each bite about 25 times. And it's important to wait a moment between bites; if you feel pressure, you should not swallow again, even if you already have food in your mouth. You'll be much better off spitting it out into a napkin than trying to swallow it.

So make sure you leave scarfing down your food in the past. Your surgeon won't leave you a whole lot of choice in the matter!

2. *Don't drink while you eat.* What we don't want you to do is make every bite of food into "soup." Say you take a bite of chicken, for example, and chase it with a small sip of water. When you chew up a piece of food *and* rinse it down with water, the food will pass through your smaller stomach faster, and your brain has less time to tell you that you're satisfied. The result is that you may inadvertently wind up eating too many calories over the course of your meal. Also

keep in mind that if your stomach is already full and you try to drink water, all you're going to do is overfill your stomach, which will cause you to throw up.

Many bypass and sleeve patients will learn early on about *dumping*, an extremely unpleasant combination of physical reactions that occurs when too much sugar or fat is consumed after surgery. If you're eating high-sugar or high-fat foods and then you rinse them down with water, you'll quicken the onset of dumping. That's why surgeons recommend that patients stop drinking about 30 minutes before a meal and do not resume until 30 minutes after. You'll learn, after a period of time, when your body is telling you that your stomach is full. So if you just adhere to the 30-minutes-before-and-after rule, you're not going to run into trouble with that water.

3. *Limit or eliminate alcohol.* There are a couple of reasons that alcohol should be avoided after surgery. First of all, alcohol is just empty calories. A calorie from alcohol is closer to the calorie content of fat than it is to protein or sugar. Secondly, alcohol tends to reduce your inhibitions, so you may become less careful about what you eat when you're drinking. And, after surgery, alcohol will hit you much harder and faster than it did before, so weight-loss-surgery patients need to be extremely cautious if they do choose to drink, and they should *never* get behind the wheel with alcohol in their system. In short, alcoholic drinks have very little nutritional value and a lot of calories, and they can make you prone to making poor or even dangerous choices. That's why we suggest that people abstain from alcohol for the first year after surgery, though we know that not everyone complies with that recommendation. There are celebrations, holidays, and other occasions when you might choose to have a drink. Surgeons aren't too worried about patients having a very occasional drink, as long as they do so safely. We're really concerned about the consumption of those empty liquid calories becoming detrimental, especially for patients who want that glass of wine every night with dinner. It's important to remember that if your consumption is limited, what you are putting into your body needs to have good nutritional value.

4. *No carbonated beverages or straws.* We've all taken a full swallow of soda and then experienced a full feeling and been forced to burp. When you take a drink of a cold carbonated beverage, all the dissolved gas in the beverage hits your warm stomach and then needs to be released. But weight-loss-surgery patients, because surgery has reduced the size of their stomachs, don't have a large reservoir to hold that gas anymore. The gas puts a lot of pressure on the new, smaller stomach, so it's going to be painful. Also, over time, the gas from carbonated beverages may actually cause the tissue of your stomach to stretch. So drinking carbonated beverages after surgery causes painful gas and can potentially make your operation less effective over time by stretching your stomach pouch. Despite these issues, patients often go on the Internet and talk to others on blogs and forums, and they read posts written by people who generally aren't following the postsurgery rules that say, *I can drink Coke. I drink carbonated stuff all the time.* But, as your surgeon will tell you, there's no nutritional value in most carbonated beverages, and drinking them may cause pain and may lead to early failure of your operation. So our recommendation is just to stay away from carbonation.

   One of the things patients often come to their surgeons complaining about is that they're gassy or feel bloated all the time. We know that, in general, you end up swallowing a lot of air when you drink with straws. That air gets into your lower intestinal tract, and you end up getting a lot more gas. Most people don't want to feel gassy, and straws will make them feel that way more often than not. That's why we suggest that patients stop using straws after surgery.

5. *Get enough vitamins, calcium, and iron.* When a surgeon either changes the size of your stomach or rearranges your intestinal tract (or both), your body's ability to absorb some vitamins and minerals is reduced. You also won't be eating as much food after surgery as you did before. Your body isn't seeing as much food or absorbing it as well as it once did, so unless the nutritional quality of your food is perfectly monitored and balanced, you're going to run into some deficiencies and will need to supplement with vitamins and minerals. Iron and calcium are not absorbed that well after surgery. Women in general have a tough time keeping bone mass on, so if

they do not supplement with calcium, they're much more susceptible to osteoporosis. We're talking about a lifelong change here; if most of the calcium in your bones is gone when you're 80, you're much more prone to fractures and other injuries.

Iron deficiency is also common after surgery, because the body doesn't absorb iron well to begin with and weight-loss surgery diverts iron away from the part of the body that absorbs it best—the duodenum, the first part of the small intestine. When you have less iron in your system, you don't make sufficient hemoglobin (the part of the red blood cell that carries oxygen), and you can become anemic. Some of the B vitamins, such as folate and B12, are also part of the production of red blood cells. The fact that iron and B vitamins aren't absorbed as well after weight-loss surgery, especially since you're not eating as much after surgery, means that you should supplement with vitamins (and maybe iron pills). A multivitamin may take care of some people's needs, but because it's difficult for the body to absorb iron, an iron supplement may be needed, especially for women of childbearing age who are still having monthly periods. Iron supplements may cause an upset stomach or lead to constipation, and they need to be taken at a separate time from multivitamins so that the two supplements don't cancel each other out. But it's a necessary inconvenience.

6. *Exercise, exercise, exercise.* There are a couple of reasons that weight-loss-surgery patients need daily exercise. Muscles burn more calories than fat, so an individual who has more muscle than fat will use more calories than a person of the same weight who has more fat than muscle. This means that a person with more muscle can afford to eat a little bit more. Exercise will also make you feel healthier and more vibrant. A body, just like a car, starts breaking down if it isn't used. Exercise can burn a few hundred extra calories a day, and the muscles you build by exercising regularly will continue to burn calories even after you've finished exercising for the day. And as you exercise and exchange body fat for more muscle tissue, you'll become more compact, because muscle is denser than fat. Most people don't care how much they weigh; they care about how big they are, and exercise helps to reshape their bodies. With regular exercise,

weight-loss-surgery patients become leaner and healthier, plus they feel better and can move freely. In addition, for people with diabetes, exercise (both aerobic exercise and strength training) helps the body use insulin better and can lower blood glucose. It's a win-win situation all around.

7. *Eat small portions and balanced meals.* One of the things that, unfortunately, we do very poorly in the U.S. is teach our kids about nutrition and appropriate eating habits. We learn from what we see at restaurants and on television—where the portions are abnormally large and have far too many calories—so we have a visual expectation of what we're *supposed* to be eating. Americans also do a poor job teaching children the importance of eating a variety of foods and including vegetables, fruits, grains, and proteins in our diets. Fast-food meals, for example, usually consist of bread, a piece of meat, cheese, and mayonnaise, and the "vegetable" is ketchup. Variety is essential so that you get the amount of fiber, the assortment of vitamins, and the right balance of protein, complex carbohydrates, and healthy fats you need to stay healthy. Having small, balanced meals and snacks during the day—unless your doctor recommends otherwise—is important so that you don't get super hungry. After surgery you should stick to one palm-sized serving of protein, 1/2 cup of starch, and one serving of fruit or vegetables per meal, plus one or two healthy snacks (a serving of fruit, vegetables, or protein) per day—unless your doctor recommends otherwise. *Tip:* Use salad plates until your portion sizes become second nature to you.

8. *No aspirin or ibuprofen and limited caffeine.* Drugs like aspirin, ibuprofen (Advil), and naproxen (Aleve)—nonsteroidal anti-inflammatory drugs (NSAIDs)—all burn the tissue of the stomach and small intestine and can cause bleeding from your gastrointestinal tract. When the size of the stomach is reduced by surgery, these drugs have to sit in a much smaller space, and they tend to drop down to the same general area in the stomach each time you take them, so the risk of developing ulcers increases. Ulcers can bleed and lead to narrowing of the connection between the stomach and the small intestine. As the body heals from an ulcer, scar tissue is

often left behind, and it can start shrinking the opening between the stomach and the small intestine. This can increase the chances of food getting stuck in the opening, and when that happens, you can run into real trouble. So we certainly don't want patients to take NSAIDs every day. If you're taking them *occasionally*, maybe once a month, or every other month, for a cold or some aches and pains, it's not going to hurt you. It's really daily use that you've got to avoid. On those occasions when you do take these medications, remember to wash the pills down with a lot of water. That will help to dilute the pills and rinse them through your new stomach. Crushing the tablets will also help. If you use liquid-gel capsules, open up the capsule and put the medication into water, yogurt, or anything that will help carry it down. But if you can get away with taking acetaminophen (Tylenol), which isn't going to burn the stomach, then that's a better option. Acetaminophen doesn't put you at the same risk, and it can be used to treat a fever, headache, or some minor muscle aches.

Here's the word on caffeine. Caffeine gives you energy by releasing hormones in your body that rev up your system. Your body wants to get going, and all of a sudden you may feel the need to look for food. The consequence of the stimulus revving up your system is that you could start to feel hungry. You may go looking for a snack, and unless you're super prepared, you probably won't be making good choices. Secondly, not everyone drinks their coffee black, and adding creamers and sugar to coffee can significantly increase the amount of calories and carbohydrate in the drink. So we certainly don't recommend that you drink *lattes* every day. Many people tend not to count liquids when tracking what they eat. They think that if it's not part of their meals, then it's not part of their calorie counts and it's okay to have. But if the coffee you drink has added sugars and creamers, you need to keep track of the calories and carbohydrates.

9. *Drink eight glasses of water a day.* Surgeons like to push water because water tends to flush out all the toxins in the body. Plus, a lot of times when we think we're hungry, we're actually thirsty, and the signals in our brains are confused. I hear all the time that when people who think they're hungry drink a glass of water, they

suddenly feel full. Bariatric surgeons recommend that patients drink eight glasses of water a day to keep the body hydrated, and flush out—especially during the weight-loss process—the toxins that your body is releasing while you're melting the fat tissue away. Drinking plenty of water will help you avoid constipation; it keeps your bowels well hydrated. One of the potential consequences of dehydration is getting kidney stones, so you really want to make sure you stay hydrated and everything gets flushed out of your system. Just remember to avoid drinking for 30 minutes before and after a meal.

10. *Eat 75 grams of protein a day.* After surgery, we want patients to eat about 1 gram of protein per kilogram of lean body mass. A kilogram is 2.2 pounds. So let's say you weigh 200 pounds. That means you would need to eat about 90–100 grams of protein a day *if* you were 200 pounds of *lean muscle*. But, if your body is half fat, you could really cut that in half. The bottom line is that we're trying to spare your muscle, so up your protein intake within reason. Your body can't manufacture all the components of protein it needs, so if you don't eat enough protein, your body has to tear down your muscles to find the building blocks it needs to create proteins to "run the machinery" in your body. We want the body to use fat—not muscle—as a source of energy. After surgery, your calories should come from proteins, complex (high-fiber) carbohydrates, and essential/unsaturated fats, in that order. If your diet consists more of protein and complex carbohydrates (like vegetables and fiber) than fat, you are going to get better nutrition than if your diet is high in fat and simple sugars and lower in protein (which is typical of the American diet and fast-food meals). So make sure you eat enough protein to spare your muscle. Plus, remember that hair and fingernails are made out of protein and your skin has a lot of protein in it, so if you are short on protein, your hair and nails will be thin and your skin is going to be dry. Looking good is as good a reason as any to keep your protein intake up! Protein shakes are part of the all-liquid post-op diet that all patients go on after weight-loss surgery. It's important to include shakes so that you can be sure to get enough protein. Even after you start eating solid foods again, we recommend keeping

protein shakes in your repertoire so that your diet doesn't fall short of necessary protein.

Some of these rules may seem extreme. But remember, we doctors didn't make up these rules for our own amusement or to make our patients miserable. We're just trying to give you all the ammunition you need to be successful on your weight-loss journey!

Consequences of Noncompliance

Occasionally, weight-loss surgery does not work as well as one would hope. Some people claim that surgery turned out to be a *temporary fix* but, in the end, *it didn't last.* Let's talk about why. In order to do that, it's important to understand what weight-loss surgery *is*—knowledge which we hope this book has helped to provide—but just as importantly, you also have to know what weight-loss surgery *is not.*

Weight-loss surgery (including gastric bypass, sleeve gastrectomy, and gastric band procedures) doesn't *make* you lose weight. By making certain changes to your anatomy, it *allows* you to lose weight. It is a tool that helps you in this struggle, a struggle that you may have had most of your life. Weight-loss surgery doesn't do the work for you. It just doesn't. If it did, we'd all be skinny forever, and I'd be out of business.

I can tell you until I'm blue in the face that weight-loss surgery calls for *a lifetime commitment and a complete change in your relationship with food.* Many patients nod enthusiastically and *seem* to get it, and most of them actually do. Some patients get caught up in the excitement of the moment; they try to absorb all the information their surgeon throws at them and end up forgetting some of it. But there are other patients who hear this information and just think, *Not me, brother.* Weight-loss surgery probably won't work for the individuals who do not want to commit to lifestyle changes.

Patients come to us with many excuses for why they cannot maintain a healthy lifestyle. Here are some examples of the excuses that we file under the category of "noncompliant":

- I have a high-stress job and I need to relax with a cocktail when I get home from work. Every day.
- The kids are running me ragged, so pizza night is a "must" for this family, including me.
- I eat out a lot and I don't want to stick out like a sore thumb because of the way I eat.
- I'm watching the game. Of course I'm going to have a beer. And chips. And whatever else I can get my hands on.
- I bruised my pinkie toe so I can't exercise.
- I don't have time to go to the gym.
- I don't have time to prepare an appropriate meal.
- A couple of diet sodas a day won't hurt me.

The list of excuses goes on and on. Weight-loss surgeons have heard them all.

The consequences of noncompliance with postsurgery lifestyle changes will quickly become evident if that's the road you choose to take. Eventually, you're going to stretch out your new stomach. You're going to undo the hunger-control mechanisms that surgery provided. You may not lose enough weight, and you won't keep off the weight you do manage to lose. If you have diabetes, your blood glucose levels may not improve sufficiently to reverse or avoid organ and nerve damage. Your blood pressure, back pain, joint pain, sleep apnea, etc.—any of the reasons you decided to have surgery in the first place—may either not improve or continue to worsen over time.

So here's a key piece of advice: If you're going to talk the talk, you've got to walk the walk. *If you're not prepared to do what is necessary to make your procedure work, then you should not have it.* Don't put your body through the stress and risk of surgery if you're unwilling to do what it takes to make the surgery successful. Please understand that this doesn't make you a bad person. It just means that you're not ready for weight-loss surgery—at least not now.

Before you opt for surgery, figure out how you got to this place. What emotional issues, painful past, or ongoing unhappiness is sending you to the drive-through every day? What fears about your future food issues are paralyzing you now? If you decide to have surgery, there are all sorts of professionals, support groups, and books out there that will help you figure out how you can learn to comply with the "rules" of postsurgery life. Take advantage of the information that is available to you and make the most of this opportunity.

The toughest step you'll take in this entire process is the first one through the door of your doctor's office. Your surgeon will provide the means for you to get and stay healthier. Having the guts to do it is all up to you.

Post-Op Changes

The sleeve gastrectomy and the gastric bypass are procedures that are designed to last a lifetime. But there still are changes that can happen after those operations that make them less effective than they were immediately after surgery.

Sleeve Gastrectomy

A sleeve gastrectomy, as we learned in Chapter 2, changes your stomach to a narrow tube, about the size and shape of a small banana, and if you are constantly trying to overfill that tube, the tube will begin to stretch out over time. That could stop and even reverse your weight loss, because you're gradually creating a bigger and bigger reservoir and putting more food into it. Could anything bad happen as the new stomach stretches? Yes, depending on which part stretches. The outer edge of the stomach, to the left of the esophagus, has a greater tendency to stretch. It's much more flexible than the other edge. So when surgeons perform a sleeve gastrectomy, we leave the inner edge of the stomach (the wall closest to the esophagus and the entrance to the small intestine) intact, and we remove the outer edge. We try to limit the flexibility of the new stomach, but patients can still stretch it out over time. The top of the stomach is more likely to stretch than the bottom, so if your stomach begins to stretch, it's possible that a little bubble will generate at the top of your sleeve. If this happens, you now have a banana-sized tube with a stretched-out bubble (usually about the size of a golf ball or bigger), and food can get trapped in that bubble. This can cause an obstruction, and you can experience reflux and regurgitation (heartburn and vomiting). On the other hand, if the whole stomach tube dilates equally all along the edge, then it allows you to eat a lot more food. When people *can* eat more food, they tend to do it, and that is how they begin to put weight back on.

All three weight-loss operations have hormonal components that help you control feelings of hunger, with the sleeve and bypass being about equal in terms of hunger control, and the band coming in a distant third. But the human body is constantly adapting. Over time your body can adjust to these hormonal changes and may no longer get the *I'm full* signal like it used to. This means that the hunger control brought on by weight-loss surgery may not be as strong or effective 5 years down the line as it was in the initial days following surgery.

The sleeve gastrectomy is still a relatively new operation without much in the way of long-term data available. So after performing a sleeve gastrectomy on a 25-year-old patient, we can't definitively tell that patient what life will be like at 40 years old, but we're pretty certain that the sleeve will be a little bit bigger and that, more than likely, *some* of the weight lost right after surgery will have been regained, but not all of it. In addition to the stomach stretching that we see in patients who over-eat after surgery, there is also some natural stretching of the sleeve that occurs. So we know that the stomach will be bigger, but what we don't know is why this sort of natural stretching affects some people more than others, and why some people have greater hunger control after surgery than others.

What has become clear is that it's not just the body's physiology that makes us eat. For example, we've all had periods of stress that affect our eating patterns. People generally tend to respond to stress in one of two ways: they either eat more during difficult times or they become stressed out and eat less. Most people who are overweight have a tendency to eat more when they're under stress. What we can say about the sleeve gastrectomy—and all of these operations, including the gastric bypass and gastric band—is that surgically created pouches (stomachs) are going to stretch a little bit over time. But we also know that when people stop looking at external portion sizes to determine how much to eat and focus instead on how they feel (by asking themselves whether or not they're experiencing hunger and if it's time to stop eating), they eat less and are satisfied.

Even more important than gaining an awareness of everything that goes into your mouth, which we certainly advocate, is learning to detect the early satiety signals (signals that tell you when you're full) that control food intake. If you think that feeling discomfort or being "stuffed to the gills" is the sign to stop eating, you're much more likely to stretch your new stomach reservoir than if you say to yourself, *I know that there's enough food in my stomach, and I should stop eating now. I'll give myself some time to let all of this food soak into my body so that I really know that I'm no longer hungry.* It's vital to learn how to tell that you're no longer hungry *before* the uncomfortable or even painful pressure of being overstuffed occurs. It's the difference between wanting food and needing food. Most people see a plate of food that tastes good and they want to finish it, even though they know that doing so could make them uncomfortable or sick. If it's going to make them feel miserable and need to lie down for an hour, they'd feel much better *not* eating too much food.

So while the smaller stomach created during a sleeve gastrectomy may stretch naturally over time, stretching that may be due to overconsumption is often avoidable. Patients who are able to differentiate between eating for hunger and eating for pleasure, out of stress, or to the point of discomfort have the upper hand in preventing excessive stretching.

Gastric Bypass

Patients who undergo a gastric bypass, the procedure that offers us the most historical data, may also have to deal with some issues as the years pass. To create the bypass, the surgeon works with the top part of the stomach, sewing a piece of intestine to a very short piece of the top part of the stomach to form a small pouch. This pouch can stretch just as the stomach can stretch after a sleeve gastrectomy. In addition, the connection—the opening between the pouch and the small intestine, called the *stoma*—can also stretch. When you eat a piece of food after a gastric bypass, it goes down your esophagus and stops in that little pouch, and it's going to sit in there until it empties through the stoma into the small intestine. When that pouch or stomach is very small, it's not very flexible; you put in a couple of bites and it's full. The stoma is very narrow, so food that's textured, rather than liquid, has to get pushed through, and this takes time. After a few years, the stomach is bigger and it's more flexible, because the body has adapted. If the opening out of it is also bigger, it can empty faster, which means that most people will be tempted to refill it quickly and more often. A few years after surgery, the rate at which a bypass patient is eating is often influenced by how quickly food can pass through their system rather than how hungry they are or how much food they think they should be eating. It's also possible that, after a bypass, the small intestine will stretch over time. It may stretch out to the size of a large stomach. The people who experience this issue can eat faster and get more calories in than they would have been able to otherwise, and, consequently, they often gain some weight.

There are other difficulties that can arise with a gastric bypass that may require surgery to fix. Some bypass patients develop what is known as a *stricture*, a narrowing of the opening between the stomach pouch and the small intestine, the stoma. Strictures can be caused by chronic irritation, and they usually occur in people who take aspirin or anti-inflammatory drugs like ibuprofen and/or are smokers. If you develop an ulcer at the stoma, scarring can occur as it heals, resulting in a narrower opening. Some patients may develop chronic ulcers because the tissue from the small intestine on the bottom side of the stoma just isn't as durable as the stomach it's connected to. This tissue from the small intestine is used to absorbing calories, not grinding food, which is what the stomach is for. Sometimes that connection between the stomach and small intestine has to be surgically redone in order to promote long-term healing.

After the stomach has been cut and separated to form the pouch for a gastric bypass, you can get what is called a *remnant stomach*. The majority of the stomach that is bypassed (meaning food no longer passes through it) is off to one side, but it can reconnect itself through a new connection called a *gastric fistula* that can form between the old stomach and the "new" one (the pouch). The end result is that food can go through the old stomach as well as the new path the surgeon has created. This can cause acid reflux and ulcers as well as weight gain.

In addition, bypass patients can get kidney stones because of the way some minerals are absorbed by the configuration of their new anatomy. Twisting of the intestines and/or bowel obstructions are also possible, but all of these things are easily fixable and do not occur too frequently. It's important to remember that these operations, despite the potential complications, are much less dangerous than staying overweight for a prolonged period of time and developing the diseases associated with chronic obesity.

One of the most common postsurgery changes for gastric bypass patients (as well as many sleeve patients) is that dumping syndrome, which is the result of eating high-fat or high-sugar foods, begins to occur less frequently. People who experienced dumping in the first year or so after surgery get a not-so-gentle reminder that there are certain foods they should not eat. But as these people start experiencing dumping less and less frequently, they realize they can eat some high-fat and high-sugar foods without getting sick, so they do. For example, if eating a cookie made a bypass patient sick after surgery but now, after some time, it doesn't, this patient may choose to eat cookies and will then be vulnerable to all the sugar and fat calories he or she has been avoiding. So while most people would be thrilled to leave dumping in the past, it's one change that can cause these operations to be less effective as time passes.

Gastric Band

Anatomically, it is *possible* that the gastric band could be initially placed in a perfect position—meaning it could, theoretically, remain perfectly configured forever. But for most patients, there are some changes that take place with their gastric band operation over the course of their lifetime. One of the more common changes is that the pouch created by the band gets a little bit bigger over time; the new stomach above the band can get one and a half to two times larger than it was when the surgeon first put the band in. Stretching of that small pouch can result from a patient putting too much food into it. The body is always adapting, so, as with other weight-loss procedures, if you constantly overfill the stomach, it may get bigger. But stretching can also happen as a natural consequence of the body adapting to the anatomical changes the operation imposes, even if what would be considered an appropriate amount of food is consumed. The body is always going to adapt to the stress caused by the restriction, so the pouch created by the band may get a little bit bigger despite the patient's best efforts and compliance with post-op rules. In addition, the pouch is located up near the diaphragm, right below an opening called the hiatus (one of the barriers that protects against acid reflux), and as that pouch enlarges, it can dilate up into the hiatus. Sometimes, after restrictive procedures like gastric banding, food can cause the new stomach to bulge into the hiatus, causing a hiatal hernia. When this happens, you can experience some sloshing of the food you eat, which can lead to reflux or indigestion.

"Learn to recognize the early signals of satiety rather than waiting until you think, *I just ate so much. I have to go lie down.*"

While it's more likely to happen if your band is too tight for too long and/or you've overfilled your stomach at most meals, everyone's pouch is going to get a little bigger over the long term. It's just your body's way of responding to a stress. If our bodies are good at anything, they're good at adapting to environmental stresses and creating new methods to deal with these stresses. If your stomach stretches a bit, it will still tell you when you're no longer hungry, but you have to learn to recognize the early signals of satiety rather than waiting until you're so full you think, *I just ate so much. I have to go lie down, or go throw up.* Unfortunately some gastric band patients tend to eat to the point where they're uncomfortably stuffed; it's as painful as being full after the biggest Thanksgiving dinner they've ever eaten, but they experience the feeling with every meal. They rely on the band's ability to inflict pain to indicate their stopping point rather than taking advantage of its ability to curb hunger earlier.

Most people are very good at eating the appropriate amount of food for the first several months after surgery; the band is new for them, and they're excited and dedicated. But then after a year or two, the novelty wears off. They start testing the boundaries, and they get a little more courageous. They realize that the pain of overeating is short-lived and is not going to kill them. Most patients adapt quickly to the uncomfortable feelings, so they're apt to overeat more often. It's not that these patients will always go to the extreme of overfilling their stomach and vomiting, but they'll try to fit in the few extra bites that they would have avoided right after the surgery. The body's long-term response to the extra food is to stretch out a little bit. It's like filling a balloon—it has a lot of elasticity at the beginning, but if you leave it overfilled for too long and then deflate it, it's not as flexible anymore. It never goes back down to the small size it was when you first tried to fill that balloon up.

If you catch overfilling early enough, your doctor can adjust the gastric band by letting some of the fluid out of the band to let food pass through your system faster. Your doctor will explain the importance of looking for loss of hunger rather than waiting for signs of discomfort to stop eating. A lot of times, if you don't leave the band overfilled too long, it will go back down to its normal size. This is one of the reasons intensive follow-ups with your doctor after surgery are so important. You can't just go to see your doctor for the first year and then avoid the doctor for the next 3 years. A lot of people want to forget where they were before surgery…and if they keep going back to their doctor all the time, it's a constant (though beneficial) reminder of where they started. Some patients would much rather just be on "autopilot" and pretend that their postsurgery body is just what they look like, and that they didn't really have to do anything special to get there. Unfortunately, this behavior can lead to higher rates of complications or weight regain.

Many times the pouch can stretch out because the opening of the band is too *small* for too long. When you have an opening that is too narrow, the area above the band can stretch out. The pouch is fairly weak and doesn't contract very well, so food tends to dwell above the band for a while before getting pushed through. Many band patients feel as though they can eat a lot, but food just doesn't pass through the band well in some cases, so the pouch muscles stretch out. When this happens, many people start having problems with reflux or regurgitation, and they subconsciously adapt to these issues by ingesting more high-calorie liquids and soft foods that melt in the mouth; these things don't require as much force to get pushed through the band as solid foods do. The problem with ingesting more liquids and soft foods is that these foods are usually not nutrient-dense and are often high in calories. Patients who eat a lot of these foods often don't feel satisfied and may gain weight. While it is possible to find softer foods that are low in calories and fat, most people, even those with the best intentions, do not choose healthy soft foods.

Not every patient is satisfied with his or her gastric band procedure. I'm often asked how many people give up on the band and have it taken out because they don't think it's worth it. In the good surgical practices it's probably about 15%, but in some practices, studies show, it can be as high as 40–50%. To put this into perspective for you, let's say you had a hip replacement. Hip replacements usually last about 10 years, so it's not surprising that many patients are back in surgery after a decade or so. Obviously, having a surgery that would last forever would be the ideal, but just because a surgery needs some maintenance definitely doesn't mean that you should regret having the surgery in the first place.

As you can see, patients may experience a variety of changes to their new anatomy over time, but the bottom line for all three of these procedures is this: weight-loss surgery, like all surgery, comes with some degree of risk. It is up to your physician and surgeon to determine if that risk outweighs the risk of staying overweight and dealing with the comorbidities—diseases such as diabetes, for example—that accompany living life overweight in the long term.

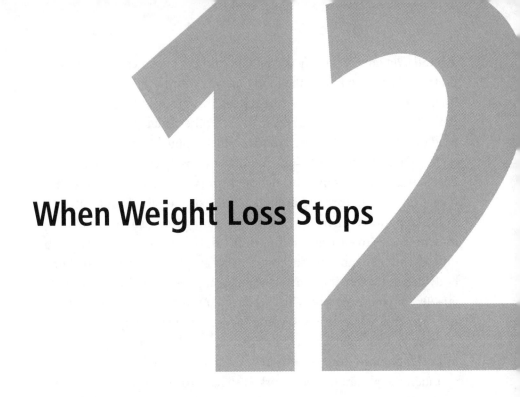

When Weight Loss Stops

Is the Honeymoon Over?

In the weight-loss-surgery community, the "honeymoon period" is that first blush of excitement postsurgery when losing weight seems effortless. A lot of people experience a honeymoon period with any new diet regime. They're excited to start it, they're excited to participate, and they see results quickly, so they're motivated. And then things slow down a little bit. When the honeymoon is over, many people want to give up. With gastric bypass and sleeve gastrectomy procedures, the honeymoon period generally lasts for the first 6 months, when you have very little hunger. It's hard for patients to eat a lot of food during this period; they have much less interest in food than they did before surgery, and they lose weight very rapidly. There are both positive and negative aspects of this rapid, easy weight loss. After about a year and a half, many patients can start eating some high-sugar/high-fat calories again—ice cream, for example, doesn't cause the same adverse reaction that it did right after surgery—so their motivation wanes, and they don't see the same dramatic weight loss they saw a year earlier. Even though you may keep losing weight, the novelty has sort of worn off at this point, and you realize,

Wow, the honeymoon really is over. Over time it becomes harder to stay on track, harder to ignore the food that was your friend before surgery. That's one of the reasons postsurgery support groups are so important. Patients in these groups can relate to each other, offer support, and keep each other motivated. These groups really become like a family.

As time goes on, weight loss eventually stops, because the body develops a new set point. Throughout history, starvation was a much bigger threat than carrying around a little extra weight. People often didn't know where their next meal was coming from, so their bodies took measures to ensure that they didn't starve. In theory, it's not much different after weight-loss surgery. You eat substantially less, and your body decides where it ultimately wants you to be—usually having lost 60–70% of your excess weight—while still protecting itself from what it may perceive as starvation. If you disagree with your body, it does things to make you comply: you get hungrier, and you're often tempted to eat more. If you don't keep your head in the game, it will be more difficult to maintain the weight loss you worked so hard to attain. There are many redundant mechanisms in the body that regulate your weight, which is why it is sometimes difficult to treat obesity with drugs. Diet drugs will generally work on *one* pathway to help you lose weight, but the body says, *Okay, but I have five other pathways. If you're going to block that one, I've got other ways to get to my goal of keeping extra energy and pounds around.* Weight-loss drugs may help a bit, but generally not enough for extremely overweight people. The body will ultimately achieve its goal (to protect you from starvation) most of the time.

Weight-loss surgeons perform procedures on tens of thousands of people, so we understand the trajectory of postsurgery weight loss. Patients tend to achieve maximum weight loss within the first 2 years of surgery, and then the average person may regain some weight. Average patients are not constantly tracking or measuring the food that's going into their mouths, they're busy living their lives, and they've become more comfortable with not thinking about food every minute.

The message to take home here is that, while maximum weight loss generally happens during those first couple of years after surgery, what you're trying to do after that is protect the weight loss you've attained. Let's say you start out with 100 pounds of excess weight and, after surgery, you lose 70 pounds. You're trying to maintain that 70-pound loss.

When you see celebrities on televison or people you know who have had weight-loss surgery, you'll see that their weight goes up and down...not all the way up to 100% weight regain, but they'll play with about 15–20% of their total weight loss. Weight-loss-surgery patients generally don't put all their weight back on after they lose it, but they tend to fluctuate around their new, lower weight; they've established a new set point. As we mentioned in Chapter 4, if you voluntarily overeat, the body wastes more calories, or if you eat too little, it starts lowering your metabolism so that you save more calories, all in an attempt to maintain your body's new set point. So it's easy to see how your weight can go back and forth a bit after surgery.

Weight Loss: Genetics vs. Environment

In order to fully understand why some people regain weight after weight-loss surgery, we need to take a look at the genetic and environmental factors that affect weight loss. There are certain aspects of weight loss that you can control consciously, but there are also "programs" that your body is running in the background that you don't have conscious control over. In Chapter 4 and earlier in this chapter we discussed that starvation was a big problem for early human beings, and that the people who ultimately survived early on were the ones whose bodies were good at preventing starvation. If we look at the development of populations who traditionally had to hunt for food, for example, we see that these people had to develop anti-starvation survival mechanisms because, in their past, there were extended periods of time when they didn't have enough food. These survival mechanisms have been passed down to us genetically and are difficult to override.

So our examination of weight loss starts with genetics, but then we need to add a cultural/environmental overlay. In the last 30 years, our genetics haven't really changed, yet we're faced with an epidemic of obesity. We are finding that environment also plays a crucial role in determining body weight. Environment refers not only to our lifestyle but also to our access to different types of foods and our expectations (from our families, restaurants, and the media) about what a meal should be. Let's think about the 1950s and what was in a TV dinner—that little tray of food defined a generation. If someone put that same tray in front of us now, most people would say, *Well, that's a nice snack, but what's for dinner?*

In general, people were a lot thinner in the 1950s because the *expectation* of what a meal should be was different. And now the food industry has figured out that what tastes good to most people is high-fat, high-sugar, very calorie-dense food, and they supply this food to us because it's their job to sell product, not protect our health. So a combination of environmental and genetic factors makes it difficult for people to continue losing weight past a certain point.

Why the Scale Won't Budge

As we learned in Chapter 4, the body defends its set point. The brain has a set point of weight or energy reserve, and weight-loss surgery allows you to move that set point to a new level, but not usually to your *ideal* weight (as dictated by insurance tables). Your body has a set weight that *it* thinks it needs to maintain, and in order to convince it to behave otherwise, you have to constantly and consciously reduce your caloric intake or do things to make your body burn more calories (such as exercising to produce more lean body mass). Translation: *you need to eat less, and move more.* Sound familiar? For most people, this is a difficult task.

When Have You Gone as Far as You Can Go?

As we discussed earlier in this chapter, usually a good rule of thumb is that patients of most weight-loss procedures have reached maximal weight loss at about 2 years. I have seen patients, however, who have spent the first couple of years after surgery just messing around, never really complying with the post-op dietary regimen, and later on down the line they decided to get serious about their weight and have somehow managed to still lose a significant amount of weight. This delayed start is certainly not behavior we recommend! But if you've gone through the program, eaten the appropriate foods, and exercised, then usually at about the 2-year mark you have figured out how much weight you're going to lose in total. With the gastric band it's about 50% of the patient's excess weight on average, if the patient is provided access to good dietitians and good psychological support. (For the places where they just put in the band, hurry you out the door, and don't really follow up with you, the results are less predictable.) Sleeve gastrectomies and gastric bypasses result in a slightly better percentage, usually about 60–70% of excess weight lost.

After the initial weight-loss period, however, the rest is really up to you. You can cheat all of these operations if you want to, and tell yourself—and everyone else—that *your* operation didn't work. Just remember that *you* have to work *with* any of these weight-loss operations in order to succeed.

At some point in your weight-loss journey, there may be a period of time when you don't lose significant weight but everything else about your body has changed. Your face may be thinner, your clothes may suddenly be too big. The body is always remodeling itself—over and over again. Lean muscle replaces fat, so if you are building muscle and losing fat, you can become smaller physically even if you're at the same weight. Building muscle can also make you feel more energetic and *younger*. So if you hit a plateau with your weight-loss, ask yourself, *How do I feel?* If the answer is, *Great,* then don't worry!

Managing Your Expectations

They say that *reality bites,* but I'm here to tell you that without a healthy serving of reality *before* you have weight-loss surgery, you're likely to be in for some real surprises. There's so much to remember before and immediately after surgery, with information coming at you from a dozen different directions, that the details of what to expect from surgery can get lost in the shuffle. A little heads-up never hurt anyone, especially when it comes to understanding and managing your expectations down the line. Here are just a few examples of the realities behind common expectations about weight-loss surgery. I'm certain you'll be able to add dozens of your own expectations to this list.

Expectation: Having weight-loss surgery will be the easy way out.
Reality: No. It takes a lifelong commitment and a complete change of lifestyle to get and keep the weight off after surgery.

Expectation: I'll fit into my skinny jeans in 6 months.
Reality: You may never fit into your skinny jeans.

Expectation: I will finally be a happy person.
Reality: Only if you have the capacity to be happy in the first place. Miserable heavy people can easily turn into miserable skinny people, and their happiness level is not always tied to just their weight. That's why pre-op education and psychological assessments as well as post-op support and, if necessary, therapy are available to help patients enjoy not only weight-loss success, but life itself.

Expectation: My friends and family will all cheer me on.
Reality: Yes, if you're very lucky. Unfortunately, many friends, family members, and significant others have trouble handling the transformation, especially if they happen to be overweight themselves.

Expectation: My type 2 diabetes will be cured!
Reality: Your diabetes will *improve*. You may actually go into remission and be able to go off your medication. While there is no cure for diabetes, you *can* slow the progression of the disease and some of its comorbidities/complications. (See Chapter 8 for more information on diabetes remission.)

Expectation: Once I've lost the weight, that's it! I'll be thin forever!
Reality: Initially, gastric bypass and sleeve gastrectomy patients frequently lose 60–70% of their excess weight, while gastric band patients lose about 50% of their excess weight. However, nothing is guaranteed to last forever. You have to work at maintaining that loss every single day (just as you would with diet and exercise alone). (*Note:* As many as 95% of people who lose weight without surgery eventually regain some or all of the weight they lose and, in some cases, gain even more weight.)

Expectation: I'm going to have the body I've wanted to have since high school.
Reality: When people lose a lot of weight in a relatively short period of time, as bariatric patients generally do, they may be left with a lot of extra skin that used to house their extra pounds. Younger patients may still have sufficient elasticity in their skin to eventually allow it to snap back into shape. For most of my patients, however, that's not the case.

While some patients choose to undergo plastic surgery (on their stomachs and elsewhere) after losing a significant amount of weight, many will opt instead for using the plethora of shaper garments available for women as well as men.

Expectation: Eventually, I'll be able to eat everything.
Reality: This is just not the case. If you figure out how to comfortably eat sushi rice or a turkey sandwich on rye after surgery (especially with a gastric band), please let us know. With each of these surgeries, there are certain foods that you'll have to strictly limit or avoid altogether.

Expectation: I'll never be able to give up soda, but how bad could it be as long as I drink diet soda?
Reality: Diet or not, the carbonation in soft drinks will stretch your pouch and cause pain, and it may lead to permanent enlargement of the new stomach, potentially allowing for significant weight gain.

Expectation: I'm going to chew everything I eat very well so I'll never throw up.
Reality: Sorry, the reality is that every once in a while something will get stuck and you'll throw up.

Expectation: If I'm not happy with the surgery, I can always go back to the way things were before.
Reality: A gastric band can be removed, but if you choose to have it removed, much of the weight you lost will likely be regained. A gastric bypass can be reversed, but only for medically necessary reasons, not just because you're tired of it. A sleeve gastrectomy is yours forever.

Expectation: I won't be hungry.
Reality: Hunger, of course, is normal, but with these operations your hunger will be satisfied with less food than it was before surgery. If you keep pushing the envelope and stuffing in more food than your new stomach is designed to hold, however, that pouch will eventually stretch. If this happens, you will be hungrier, and you will no doubt end up eating more.

Expectation: I will live longer than I would have without the surgery. **Reality:** Yes, there is a chance you will live longer because, by having weight-loss surgery, you're probably taking most of the comorbidities (diseases associated with long-term, unchecked obesity) out of the equation—or greatly improving any comorbidities you already have.

Establishing a New Relationship with Food

When you opt for weight-loss surgery, your life will change because your *lifestyle* will change—how you eat, what you eat—your entire relationship with food changes. Weight-loss surgery does not "work" all by itself—*you* have to make it work. And it's a *lifetime* commitment. So think about it carefully before making the decision to have surgery. The consideration of this commitment is as important as the decision to have the surgery itself. I'm a surgeon; I love doing these operations and making significant changes in people's lives. But you've got to meet me halfway and run with your new lifestyle. And one of the most important steps in adjusting to a postsurgery lifestyle is establishing a new relationship with food. There are a number of things that patients need to learn how to manage after surgery, including how to eat, how to get their bodies back to a healthy state, and how to maintain good health. Hopefully, a good educational program will be available to you—and required—prior to surgery to help you manage these things.

So many of today's popular diet programs have someone else planning all your meals for you and giving you premeasured portions. These kinds of programs ask you to pick one from column A and one from column B and eat these meals three times a day. People using these diet programs may not be learning what the nutritional content of the food is or how to make proper food choices. Part of what you get from a good presurgery program is a basic nutritional education; even something as simplistic as learning to identify carbohydrate, fats, and proteins is beneficial. Having sample diets can be very helpful, but in our society, you still have to be able to make choices. People need to learn how to read labels—bariatric surgeons stress that—so they actually know what's in the foods they purchase and eat. After surgery, patients aren't just handed a box of proportioned food and told to eat it. Luckily, I think that the hunger-supressing effects of weight-loss surgery actually encourage a lot of people to read nutrition labels. If you don't feel as if you're starving all the time, and you aren't just putting something in your mouth because you need to, you'll probably read the label a little more carefully and take the time to decide whether or not a food is a great choice. So I think surgery allows you to actually think about what you're eating, whereas before surgery you may not have been thinking, just consuming automatically.

So much eating is done on autopilot in our society today. We eat because it's 7 A.M. and we think it's time to eat, because we're watching television, or because the game is on and we see that hamburger commercial again. Unfortunately, we do have a lot of social expectations about food that have been developed or culturally passed down to us. So someone may be telling you when you should eat breakfast, lunch, and dinner. For example, you may remember being told, *You should be hungry at 6 P.M. because that's when I'm making dinner,* or *You need to finish what's on your plate, you're wasting food and there are people starving in other countries.* Americans are also eating out *a lot*. In restaurants, we're given portions that should feed multiple people rather than a single person, and we've come to think that's how much we're supposed to eat. When people get serious about a postsurgery lifestyle, I think they learn that the portion sizes needed to maintain their weight are much smaller than they ever imagined.

Surgeons and physicians sometimes run into family members of weight-loss-surgery patients who are worried that the patient is not eating enough. We explain that we've checked the patient's labs and he or she is nutritionally replete, meaning protein levels and vitamin levels are all great, and the patient is maintaining a healthy weight and eating enough. Sometimes the family member just *thinks* that the patient needs to eat more. And that's *their* problem. This may be a cultural thing; in a lot of cultures eating food that someone has prepared is a sign of respect and love. People think, *If you don't eat my food, you don't love me.* And in these cultures, if people come over, you can't let anyone go hungry, so you make enough food for an army. Some patients experience a lot of cultural pressure to eat.

I think for a lot of people, satisfying their hunger is different from eating until they feel stuffed. However, many people think they should feel stuffed after every meal, and they're not going to get that stuffed feeling unless they overeat greatly. I've heard people say that it's not Thanksgiving unless they have to unbutton their pants afterwards—but some people feel that they should be doing that after every meal. Obviously, this is not something that I'd advise, especially for people who have had weight-loss surgery.

So how much should a weight-loss-surgery patient know about proper nutrition? A lot! The more you know, the better choices you'll make, the more variety you'll discover, and the greater your success following surgery will be. (Many of my own patients report that their newfound knowledge of nutrition has made their families better eaters. They may be surprised…but I'm not!)

However, there's no getting around the fact that there will be things you have to give up after surgery. The patients who do best, the ones we surgeons can help the most, are the ones who come to us for medical reasons. When patients come in strictly for the cosmetic benefits of weight loss, it's generally harder to convince them to give up certain things in their lives. Most people come see a bariatric surgeon because they have diabetes or high blood pressure, they've had a heart attack, or they need to have knees or hips replaced, and their health has really confronted them with a choice: lose weight or live with the worsening consequences. These patients usually realize that they'll experience continued deterioration for the rest of their lives if they continue on this course. Many of them will say, *The party's over,* and trade the decadence of their former life for a lot more vibrancy, much better health, and a better quality of life. They've had enough experience and been confronted with enough adversity to see the consequences of being overweight as a reality rather than just something they've heard or read about. We grow up hearing that if we don't brush our teeth, they are going to fall out. It's hard to visualize that when you're 10 years old, but when you're 40 years old and you've had a couple of root canals, it's easier to see how important good dental care is. Luckily, most of our patients have had enough life experience to see that there's a give-and-take involved in almost everything, so the majority of them are willing to sacrifice at least a little to get the considerable benefits of weight-loss surgery.

> **"The hotter your body is running, the more fuel it's burning…it's burning fuel even when it's idling."**

Giving up on overeating is difficult for many people, especially those who describe themselves as "volume eaters"—those who eat abnormally large portions out of habit or because the need for the emotional comfort they receive from eating copious amounts of food is often confused with physical hunger. But it is essential for people with unhealthy eating habits to change their relationship with food after surgery. The bottom line is simple: if you're not losing weight, you're consuming too many calories. Because of the way the energy equation works, in order to lose weight you have to take in less energy than you need to maintain your current weight. Muscle tissue burns more calories than the more inert tissues, such as fat, so the more muscle you have, the more calories you'll need to maintain your body. The hotter your body is running, the more fuel it's burning. And just like a hot rod, it's burning fuel even when it's idling. Exercise helps burn calories and helps develop more muscle mass, which in turn burns more calories. Looked at another way, some people (especially those with less muscle mass) need fewer calories to maintain their bodies at rest, so you can't just look at the person's plate next to you in a restaurant and say, *She's skinny; if she can eat that much, I should be able to eat that much and maintain a healthy weight.* Not everyone metabolizes food the same way.

It is extremely important for everyone, especially weight-loss-surgery patients, to figure out the difference between not being hungry and being full. The magic word we use is *satiety*, which means *satisfaction with your state*. If you aren't satisfied, then you're hungry. But satiety is a different feeling from being stuffed. Ideally, you really want to stop eating when your hunger is gone; you don't want to continue eating until you feel like you've just had Thanksgiving dinner (even on Thanksgiving).

For a lot of people, hunger—that insatiable desire to seek out food when your body is telling you it has to be fed—dissipates within about 15 minutes of eating. Bariatric surgeons try to get people to differentiate between feeling stuffed, which most people mistake for being full, and being satisfied, that is, no longer hungry. Unfortunately, when it comes to satiety signals, there are no flashing yellow lights to say CAUTION or red lights to say STOP. It's one of the reasons we ask you to take a pause, take a time-out, take a break after half an hour of eating to let your body catch up rather than eating continuously for 2 hours. Many times this pause will help you realize that you're not eating because you're hungry, you're eating because you're bored, or because everybody else is eating, or because it tastes good and it's *there*. Sometimes people get so full that they're stuffed and ready to throw up, but they'll still try to stick one more bite into their mouths. It's not hunger that is pushing them to eat at that point; and that's what we try to get people to understand as they adjust to their new eating patterns after surgery.

Some patients pine for that volume, those big plates of delicious food. Well, you're still going to be able to enjoy food. Delicious food. Just not as much of it as you did before surgery. You will soon learn to make good use of doggie bags so you'll be able to enjoy your favorite foods again for dinner the next day and maybe even for lunch the day after that. Your food choices should become healthier, too, as you begin to lose weight, because you won't want to sabotage your own efforts.

Food will still be delicious, but after surgery it probably won't be as important in your life as it once was. One of my patients, whose social engagements always revolved around getting together with friends for meals, told me that her new mantra is, *It's not the food, it's the company.* And while it may have taken a little getting used to, she is now enjoying herself as much as she ever did. She just makes different choices.

One of the most difficult eating habits to break is what we call *mindless eating*: finding your hand in a bag of chips, a box of cookies, or a bowl of nuts without really noticing how much you're eating. One strategy to avoid mindless eating is to get into the practice of measuring out those "mindless" snacks and putting them in a cup, so that you actually have an end to the serving. It's much like when people want to establish good sleeping habits. If you put a television in your bedroom and you jump into bed and watch it, you might have problems with insomnia because now your bed represents entertainment, and there are no longer defined limits between places of entertainment and places of rest. The same thing is true with food; you don't want to eat a whole bag of chips, so the last thing you should do is put the entire bag on your lap and mindlessly eat while you're distracting yourself with television. You want to create a very well-defined place to eat. I recommend that you sit down at the table and impose a time constraint or a structure on your eating. For example, plan for a meal or snack to last no longer than 30 minutes. Most people are no longer hungry after about 15 minutes; they generally just eat for taste or out of habit after that, so you want to minimize the distractions when you're eating. The television is the biggest culprit when it comes to mindless eating, of course, because it's easy to just put things in your mouth without thinking about it while you're enjoying a show. You want to make eating its own activity and make sure it's associated with hunger. It's all a matter of keeping your head in the game, making good choices, and taking responsibility for what, when, and where you eat.

Nobody said that changing your relationship with food after surgery was going to be easy as pie (oh, sorry, poor choice of words). You've got to *really* want it. You've got to learn how to recognize when you're no longer hungry. And you've got to be willing to give up the comfort of eating whatever you want, whenever you want (often for the wrong reasons), in favor of living a better and, in all probability, longer life.

Revision and Conversion Surgery

A couple of words are starting to float around the medical community about re-operations or surgical corrections performed on weight-loss surgeries. One of those words is *revision,* and it's even starting to show up on billboards and in television and newspaper ads. The term *revision* usually means repairing an operation. So for gastric band patients, for example, if a band has a pouch that has become dilated, we can move the band up to re-create a small pouch again. If a piece of the band is broken, we'll repair that piece. For the gastric bypass patient whose pouch has increased in size, we can reconfigure the pouch or correct any connections that are allowing food to travel through too quickly.

Another term we're hearing more and more these days, which should not be confused with revision, is *conversion,* which means actually changing from one type of weight-loss operation to another. For example, let's say the stomach pouch created by your weight-loss surgery has become enlarged. Now you can eat larger volumes of food, and you do because your hunger isn't controlled effectively anymore. It's unclear whether just returning the pouch and/or any enlarged connections to normal size is going to give you enough help if you've put on a significant amount of weight. So unless there was something grossly abnormal with the mechanisms for weight loss provided by the initial surgery, usually just making minor changes isn't going to be enough. If you had your initial operation 10 years ago and it's only now showing some minor changes, that indicates that the body has been smart enough to adapt, and it may be time to create an additional weight-loss mechanism—by trying a different operation to help you lose weight again.

With the gastric bypass, if the pouch has stayed pretty close to the size it was immediately after surgery and you are eating correctly but are still not losing weight, another mechanism allowing greater malabsorption of calories can be added in order to kick-start weight loss. The surgeon can accomplish this by moving the bottom connection of the bypass a little bit further downstream, so that less of your intestine is able to participate in the absorption of nutrients and calories. For a gastric bypass, revision of the original surgery is often the best option.

On the other hand, with a gastric band, because it's only encircling the stomach, and it has the weakest physiologic effects of all the weight-loss surgeries for most people, converting it to either a sleeve gastrectomy or a gastric bypass is a good option to add additional weight-loss measures or even to help you maintain the weight you've already lost. If you have a gastric band and you feel hungry all the time, if you find yourself white-knuckling it to maintain the weight loss, or if you've put 10 pounds back on and you know 20–30 more pounds are on the way, then we need to add those additional surgical mechanisms in order to help you maintain the weight loss that the initial operation gave you.

It's still unclear how to best fix a sleeve gastrectomy, the newest of the weight-loss procedures available. Sleeves will dilate over time, and certain parts of the stomach are more likely to stretch than others, so one of the things that people can develop in the long term with a sleeve is a little bubble at the top of their sleeve that can lead to reflux. If what you're trying to correct is chronic reflux, food getting stuck, or regurgitation, just revising the sleeve for that is possible and reasonable without fundamentally changing the mechanism. If patients are looking to restart weight loss after regaining weight with the sleeve, they can either convert the procedure to a gastric bypass or, less likely, opt for one of the more severe malabsorptive operations such as a duodenal switch or biliopancreatic diversion (try saying that three times fast!). If, down the line, we find that a lot of people with sleeve gastrectomies end up regaining a significant amount of weight (and diabetes develops or worsens because of it), there will no doubt be more conversions as sleeve patients' bodies adapt to the initial surgery over time.

Having a revision or conversion surgery doesn't mean that you have failed or that your initial surgery has failed. It's akin to having a knee replacement or a hip replacement and finding that, 10 years later, it's not as strong as it was when you first had it done. That replacement may be worn out, and you may decide to get a new replacement put in. You wouldn't call that a failure of the first replacement, you've just hit the limit of what that first operation can do for you, and now it's time to re-establish the mechanism in order to get you moving again. Weight-loss surgery progresses in much the same way; sometimes surgical interventions are necessary.

Although the sleeve hasn't been around long enough to make similar assertions, we do know that you can have eventual weight regain with the gastric bypass—significant weight regain in 15–20% of the patients over the long term. While that means 80–85% of the people are doing great, about 15% of bypass patients may *not* enjoy fantastic long-term results. Unless something grossly abnormal took place during the initial surgery that needs to be repaired, most of the time your surgeon will need to add a different mechanism to help you achieve extra weight loss. Weight-loss surgery really works by controlling your hunger and making you satisfied with less food, but a lot of the surgical mechanisms aren't just mechanical, they're physiological and hormonal in nature. And sometimes what you need to do is shake up the system and create a new set of mechanisms to restore the physiology that you got from the original operation.

It's hard to say what percentage of people will eventually require a second surgery (or to predict with certainty which weight-loss procedure will work best for each individual patient). It has a lot to do with the patient's age, genetics, and general health at the time of the first surgery. What many of us in the field see as the eventual best-case scenario for successful patient weight loss is a combination of drug therapy and surgery; this is what we're hoping for. Well, that and an unequivocal way to determine which operation is going to work best for each patient. Surgeons certainly have patients who have had the simplest weight-loss procedure—the band—and done very well. They keep all the weight off, their hunger is satisfied, and 10 years out, the initial surgery is still all they need. These patients never needed a second, bigger operation and, perhaps, they never will. But, as we've already mentioned, there is also a group of people for whom the band doesn't last as long as we would like. If we had the ability to say to these patients, *Okay, your genetic fingerprint indicates that you're not going to do great with the band, you'll do much better with a bypass,* or *We can predict that if you have a gastric band put in, you'll eventually need one of the stronger operations,* then that's what we would do, so you'd only need to have one surgery. But that just isn't possible at this point. We do know that there is no perfect operation right now, so it may turn out to be an operation plus an appetite suppressant that gives you the magic formula to improve your illnesses, help you lose all of the weight you need to lose, and keep the weight off forever. I think we're going to see more and more of this kind of treatment combination in the future rather than relying on surgical revisions and conversions to help patients to keep all the weight off.

"We're currently seeing about 15–20% of patients over the long term coming in for a revision or 'tune-up.' "

Revisions exist primarily for two reasons. First, they are used to treat complications for people who have reflux or difficulty eating because their surgical connections are getting narrower or their pouches are enlarging. Secondly, they help to prevent weight regain. So the decision about whether to pursue a revision or a conversion depends on what you're trying to accomplish with the second surgery. We're currently seeing about 15–20% of patients over the long term, across the board, coming in for a revision or "tune-up." This certainly isn't the end of the world. We also need to remember that there are a lot of benefits derived from losing a significant amount of weight and maintaining that weight loss for a number of years. So the need for a second surgery should not be viewed as a failure. We have to remind ourselves that obesity is a chronic disease, and most patients are in store for a lifelong battle against it and the illnesses that accompany it. Improved health is attainable with these operations.

Weight loss is incredibly difficult. Even with behavioral therapy and meal replacements, most people will not maintain the weight loss long-term. However, healthful eating and physical activity have their own benefits, independent of weight, particularly in people with diabetes. But weight-loss surgery definitely makes sense for people looking for long-term weight loss because it consistently works for most patients.

Think about this: We all know people who have had heart surgery, either having stents placed or undergoing bypass grafting, in order to get their hearts running again. Would these heart-surgery patients say that they never would have had the surgery if they knew it would fail after 10 years? Would they say they regret the operation since they *only* got 10 years out of it? Probably not. The illnesses that accompany long-term, unchecked obesity are chronic diseases, such as diabetes, so needing multiple surgical interventions over a long period of time doesn't condemn the original procedure. But knowing that one surgery isn't necessarily a cure-all should make patients want to do everything they can to prolong good health, which means buying into the whole package—changing your eating habits, eating healthy and being vigilant about what you should and should not eat, and exercising and moving regularly.

So you shouldn't feel bad if you require a revision or conversion surgery. Success is all about managing and keeping your expectations realistic. Let's say you initially had 100 pounds of excess weight and, 2 years later, you're 70 pounds down. If, 10 years later, you still have 50 pounds off, if your diabetes, hypertension, and cholesterol levels are still much better off than they were before surgery, and if it's much easier for you to walk even though you're older, then you're still *successful*. You don't necessarily need to achieve maximum weight loss to have a good quality of life. However, if you find your blood glucose levels are creeping up or your blood pressure is up and you have more chronic diseases that would benefit from extra weight loss, then a revision or conversion is reasonable; you're simply mounting a new offensive against the enemy we were trying to attack in the first place. Bariatric surgeons are here to correct your health, not just make you fit into a smaller pair of pants.

Regaining Weight

The majority of people don't regain much weight after weight-loss surgery, though I acknowledge that *much* is a relative term. Your weight may fluctuate—overall you could regain around 15–20% of your total weight loss—but even if you veer off the path of appropriate foods and are not as vigilant as you were right after surgery, you're probably not going to gain all of the weight back. However, you should develop good eating habits up front, because it's easier to be committed from the outset than to break bad habits later on. Of course, there will always be those people who say, *Let's take this operation out for a spin and see what it can do on its own. I can always commit and make lifestyle changes somewhere down the line.* But you're much better off "driving" your operation carefully right from the start.

Weight-loss surgery sometimes gets a bad rap from habitual naysayers, but most patients will still have a significant amount of weight off 3–5 years after surgery. With a gastric band, patients are generally at about 40–50% of excess weight lost in that time frame, with bypass and sleeve patients at about 50–60% of excess weight lost. That is not to say, of course, that weight-loss-surgery patients don't gain weight; as we've seen, some do put on weight for a variety of reasons.

Gastric bypass patients may begin to regain weight a while after surgery because they were dependent on dumping syndrome (the uncomfortable consequence of eating high-fat and/or high-sugar foods) following surgery to help them stay away from certain foods. If the discomfort of dumping was the only thing keeping some patients away from those unhealthy foods, then when the dumping eventually lessens or goes away, as it does for many bypass patients after a couple of years, you'll see these people start to gain weight back as they reintroduce foods that are high in fat, sugar, and calories into their diets.

"Whichever surgical option you choose, there can be a combination of circumstances that sabotages your long-term weight maintenance."

There are more long-term results for the bypass than the sleeve gastrectomy right now, but doctors who have been performing weight-loss surgeries for a long time think that patients are going to see more weight regained with the sleeve gastrectomy than the gastric bypass 5 years down the line because the gastric bypass procedure appears to deliver more hunger-controlling hormonal changes than the sleeve does. When gastric band patients (and their doctors) become complacent and don't manage the band well, then patients are more likely to gain weight. A surgeon can tell patients not to eat fast and not to stuff themselves, but if they constantly push the envelope a little bit, then the body is going to adapt in size and capacity to what it's being fed, and weight gain will be the result.

Whichever surgical option you choose, there can be a combination of circumstances that sabotages your long-term weight maintenance. After a period of time, the operation may no longer give you the ability to take in an appropriate amount of calories—to regulate your caloric intake—so you feel hungry again and, consequently, you gain weight. When this happens, we take a look at the patient's current anatomy, and we may find that either the stomach has gotten bigger or the opening out of it is huge. The body has adapted by stretching; now the patient can shovel the food in, and there's no stopping it. Maybe they are drinking their calories by indulging in a lot of milkshakes from their favorite fast-food restaurant, or maybe they're eating any tasty food that will go down. Some patients have a problem with grazing—eating small amounts of food throughout the day. No matter how it's done, eating more calories causes weight gain.

But then there are patients who come in and their anatomy is completely normal; they have a small stomach and a small opening, but somehow they're getting more calories in. Some patients have been following all the rules since their surgery, but after a few years they begin to feel hungrier, so they start to eat more than they should. As we mentioned in Chapter 11, the hunger-controlling hormone changes brought on by surgery can become less effective over time. Your body decides that it's not going to give a hunger-suppression or satiety signal—at least not as strongly as it did right after surgery. If the brain doesn't get that signal, it will take more food for you to be satisfied. You'll keep eating until you get that signal, rather than adhering to the portion control rules that allowed you to take the weight off initially. Eating a few hundred calories more than your body needs a day can add up to a weight gain of about 10 pounds a year; that's 100 pounds in 10 years!

So a few years after surgery, some people begin to eat more food, either because they've lost the physical restriction from surgery or because the hunger-controlling hormone changes that their surgery accomplished just don't do it for them anymore. However, it's not always the *volume* of food a patient is eating that's the problem; sometimes patients gain weight because they start eating the wrong *type* of food. Right after surgery, gastric bypass and sleeve gastrectomy patients are told to eat 75 grams of protein every day. If they eat other foods—like the high-fat, high-sugar foods that made them overweight in the first place—they won't be able to get the protein in that they need. But usually at some point on their journey, the patient's belief that only *healthy foods* should go into their body diminishes, or the resolve to eat healthy weakens. Whereas right after surgery they looked for high-protein, low-fat foods that are high in complex carbohydrate, now they're just not satisfied with those foods. Eating becomes more of a recreational activity again, and this can certainly lead to weight gain.

Regaining weight can be incredibly frustrating, much like a computer crash. That's why we tell patients to start the process over. First, find out if there is any physiological reason that weight is being regained. If so, talk to your health-care team and fix it! If not, you may need to examine your current eating habits, one by one, and make any necessary adjustments. (Ask yourself, for example, *How did those cookies get into my pantry?*) Maybe go back to drinking protein shakes once or twice a day, eating healthy meals, and keeping "legal" snacks on hand. Or join/rejoin a support group. Let your surgeon handle the physiology; you take care of the psychology and eating behaviors. The mechanism for success is already there. Sometimes you just need to flip the switch and reboot.

Making the Most of Your Environment— and the People in It

One of the most important aspects of attaining and maintaining a healthy weight after weight-loss surgery is the attitude of the people around you, and your attitude toward them. There are going to be difficult days. You have to change your eating habits, and if people are always being critical of you, or even criticizing what you've achieved, it can be very stressful. Many patients aren't self-confident enough to ignore negative people. Hopefully, you'll have people around you who will help you not eat that extra cookie, or will encourage you to not even bring cookies into the house. If you're lucky, maybe you'll have someone who will even give up cookies themselves to support you. It's important for people to be supportive and not *diminish* your accomplishments. A positive environment is much more beneficial for patients than a negative one.

Manage Your Environment

We've all heard the adage *food is love*. Many of our patients have taken that adage to the extreme before surgery, and it ended up getting them into trouble. Some patients are used to taking care of other people, and that includes feeding them. And the caregiver mentality prevents these people from putting themselves at the top of their own priority list.

Surgeons heartily recommend that you try to climb that totem pole at home and make yourself a higher priority so that you can become healthy enough to take care of your family. Manage your own environment so that your food needs are accommodated, regardless of what everyone else eats. Plan your meals ahead of time, and keep healthy snacks readily available. Ask the family to either let you know when those healthy items are running low, if they share them, or ask them to lay off your stash altogether. You don't want to be stuck at 10:00 P.M. with only a bag of chocolate chip cookies staring you in the face. One of my patients went to the length of slapping sticky notes on her snacks that said "Mom." It worked!

Don't forget to count your workplace as part of your environment when it comes to food. If you work in one of those offices where cupcakes appear for every special occasion (even if the occasion is simply that it's Friday), you can try to change the culture of the office, but you can't count on having much success with that. So make up your mind not to indulge. *At all.* Have your own snacks on hand to get you through the tough moments, and you can feel quietly superior when you walk by those cupcakes!

Personal Relationships

When it comes to personal relationships, many weight-loss-surgery patients may have relationships that are codependent. People with weight issues may lack self-confidence and feel as if they are settling for the person they are with because they can't do any better, or they may be staying in a relationship in order to be taken care of. Some spouses may actually sabotage their partner's weight-loss efforts for fear of either not being needed anymore or becoming less desirable as their significant other's weight is coming off, and he or she starts looking and feeling better and getting more attention than before. This disruption in the relationship's dynamic can throw a postsurgery patient for a loop. That's why it is so important to have people to share things with, both positive and negative things. After surgery, it's time to circle the wagons and make sure you have a solid support system in place.

Adjusting to Your New Body and Lifestyle

Weight-loss-surgery patients react in a variety of ways to substantial weight loss. While most people like the attention and enjoy feeling better and looking better, there will always be those who will privately hold on to their previous identity as an overweight person in terms of body image. That image doesn't always change along with physical appearance when they look in the mirror. That's one of the reasons carefully choosing which family members and friends you spend time with is so important. Talk to the people closest to you about your journey. But don't be surprised if some people are rather judgmental, especially after you begin to lose significant weight. They may even try to consciously or unconsciously sabotage your efforts. These are the folks who should be taken in small doses until you become more confident and comfortable with your new body.

One of the commitments you'll need to make after surgery will be to engage in some form of regular exercise. Enlist a friend or group of friends to go with you. Find something that's fun for you, and make it a regular part of your lifestyle. If no one will go with you, go anyway! Meet new people—gym buddies—and share support for each other's efforts. Keep to a regime. You'll be surprised how much faster half an hour of cardio passes when you can chat with a pal.

We've mentioned this before, but it bears repeating: Find a support group in your area through your doctor's office or hospital and/or join an online discussion where you can share your ideas and concerns, as well as pick up pointers from people who have been there. I've had patients join groups for certain weight-loss programs, even if their surgery doesn't allow them to follow that program to the letter, just so they can regularly touch base with other people who require vigilance to maintain their weight. It's the *awareness* and support that are important.

Don't shrink from socializing with friends, even if it means eating in restaurants. Just check out the menu ahead of time to make sure your selections are appropriate and easy, especially in the early stages following surgery. You can find something you can eat at most restaurants, especially if you take a sneak peek at the menu—many restaurants have menus available online. Making your selections in advance will help you avoid surprises and temptations when you get to the restaurant. You may find that appetizers will be the right fit for you in terms of portion size. You can ask to have an appetizer brought to you when the others get their meals. Otherwise, if you order a full entrée, ask for a doggie bag right away and pack up at least half of your meal so that you won't be tempted to overeat. Just know you're going to have a great lunch the next day while the others are settling for peanut butter and jelly.

Weight-loss surgery isn't meant to be punitive. It certainly shouldn't isolate you from family, friends, or workmates or keep you from attending any event of your choosing. Enjoy socializing with others as often as possible, especially those who are supportive of your journey, but try to adopt a new attitude about social gatherings and dining out. As my patient who created a new mantra for herself when it came to dining with friends would say: "It's not the food, it's the company." Put that mantra to work for you!

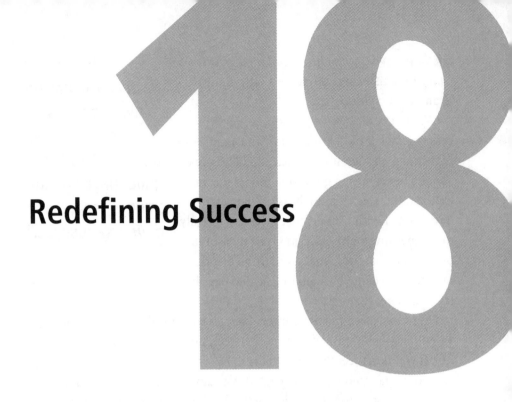

Redefining Success

What exactly is *success* when it comes to weight-loss surgery? There are plenty of patients who believe they have not attained success unless they have lost 100% of their excess weight. These patients may be in for a lifetime of frustration. Surgeons have a different measure of success. Gastric bypass and sleeve gastrectomy patients often initially attain weight loss of 60–70% of their excess weight, and gastric band recipients see around 50% of their excess weight lost much of the time. When it comes to weight loss, this is success.

In addition, what I love to see are patients whose blood glucose numbers drastically improve, whose knees and hips stop "screaming" on a daily basis, and whose blood pressure and cholesterol readings return to the normal range—the patients who will now live longer and better lives having been relieved of the stress that unchecked obesity puts on the body. This is part of the criteria by which I measure success, in addition to the above statistics provided to us by the American Society of Metabolic and Bariatric Surgery purely for weight loss.

So if you are a patient with diabetes, ask yourself, *How's my A1C?* Is it below 6%? That's success. *How's my blood pressure? How's all that joint pain?* Better? These are also measurements of success. *And how is my doctor behaving when he sees all these positive changes?* Satisfied (and maybe a little smug)? Yeah, that's *definitely* success.

When it comes to weight-loss surgery, success is growing old with and *for* your family. It's living long enough for your kids to take care of *you*. It's being such a good role model for them that your teenagers actually ask if they can have a salad with dinner; that means you really did something right. Success is not measured by your belt size. It's what's under the belt that matters, especially if it's no longer that beer belly that can so easily translate into a heart attack.

How else is weight-loss-surgery success measured? Well, in Chapter 14 we talked about the difference between not being hungry and being full. If you don't feel the need to finish every morsel of food on your plate anymore, that qualifies as success. If you can truly enjoy the food that you *are* eating rather than missing the food you are *not* eating, that's a huge step toward long-term successful weight loss. And, of course, if you don't treat every special occasion—Thanksgiving, Mother's Day, Fourth of July, Groundhog Day—as an excuse to stuff yourself, you'll be way ahead of the game.

With a little practice after surgery, you'll remember to take a time-out during your meal to let your body catch up, knowing that your body needs about 15 minutes to let you know if you're really still hungry (and more often than not you won't be). You'll feel satisfied with less food— not *deprived*, but *satisfied*. Success can be measured when you create new eating patterns by just listening to your body, which, by the way, won't always be saying *I'm starving! Feed me!*

Success is also attained when you manage to get off the couch and into the gym…or onto a hiking trail, or you go on a walk around the block. Anything that keeps you moving will help keep you off those shopping scooters at the supermarket. Movement begets more movement and weight loss. I'm not saying you have to love it, I'm just asking you to do it. Regular exercise is necessary for achieving and maintaining weight loss.

Success is the need to have your driver's license picture retaken because you're tired of getting stopped by airport security for not looking like your presurgery photo. It's those *oh my goodness!* moments when you run into old friends who haven't seen you in a while. It's pulling out a favorite jacket from the back of the closet and finding that it belongs in the charity pile with the rest of the clothes that are swimming on you now.

Most of all, success is defined by how you feel about the person looking back at you in the mirror every day. Whether or not you look exactly the way you thought you would, whether or not those skinny jeans from high school are still on the shelf in the closet, whether you have more money, more romance, or more of whatever other people use to define as success, you need ask yourself how you *feel* compared to before. If you feel better, then you've succeeded. *You* are the one who counts.

Keeping Your Head in the Game: Making Weight Loss Last

If I wanted to make this the shortest chapter in the book, I could sum up my advice on how to make weight loss last in just four words: *It's up to you*. In order to get a better idea of how to make your weight-loss procedure as effective as possible in the long run (and maximize your weight loss), let's recap some of what you've read over the course of this book and combine it with information you've probably been gathering for a long time from your experience trying to lose weight on your own.

First of all, bariatric surgeons give you the *tool* to make significant, permanent, life-changing weight loss possible. However, even the best tool won't work if you never take it out of the box, and neither will this one. Your surgeon and physician can't go home with you, shop for you, prepare meals for you, or sit there and watch you eat. Surgery takes care of the physical part. The emotional part and the psychological part, those are on you. If you're ready to take that responsibility and do the hard work that comes with it—to change the way you think, feel, and behave toward food—then you and your surgeons can make a good team. If you're not there yet, that's okay. We're not going anywhere.

You need to understand that there will be certain things you'll have to give up, and these things differ a little bit depending on which procedure you have done. For all three weight-loss procedures, you have to give up eating large portions and doing so at unregulated speeds. That's *for sure*. You just can't eat that way after surgery. If you try to do it, you're going to be awfully uncomfortable. That goes for the gastric band, the gastric bypass, and the sleeve gastrectomy. You also need to give up things that are going to sabotage your weight-loss efforts, so high-calorie liquids, refined carbohydrates, and fatty foods have to be extremely limited. Gastric band patients especially won't lose weight if they subsist on high-calorie liquids.

"You need to give up things that are going to sabotage your weight-loss efforts."

With the gastric bypass and, to a lesser extent, the sleeve gastrectomy, patients can experience that really unpleasant, adverse reaction to the wrong foods known as *dumping*. It kind of feels like a cross between hypoglycemia (low blood glucose) and a panic attack, and sometimes involves cramping, vomiting, and diarrhea. It's an altogether unpleasant experience. And while each episode of dumping passes fairly quickly, patients may experience dumping frequently for the first couple of years after surgery. So, in order to avoid dumping, you'll need to give up ice cream, cookies, cakes, and candies. These foods should already be history for people with diabetes, but we know that's not always the case. This is the time to really commit to making the choice to be healthier; anything more than a taste of these foods will result in real discomfort.

Adverse reactions to specific foods can also occur with the gastric band, because when you reach a level of tightness with the band that works for you, it may be too tight for you to eat some foods comfortably. For example, gastric band patients can pretty much forget about eating the bread from a sandwich. If you took sourdough bread, sliced it really thin, and toasted it, it may be okay, because then it's crunchy and less likely to get stuck in the band. But just eating a piece of bread is not such a good idea. I once got a call from a patient who had been in bed all weekend from pain caused by one bite of a Hawaiian roll. That won't be on her menu again anytime soon. Anything gummy and/or sticky, like sushi rice, and anything with a lot of gluten (if it doesn't contain a lot of fat to make it slippery) can plug up the small opening left by the band, so you have to give up those things. But for the most part, you'll be able to find foods you can eat—specific things that work for you. For example, you don't necessarily need to avoid *all* bread products with a gastric band. Wheat crackers are crunchy and they can contain complex carbohydrates, so they are not a bad choice. There's just going to be a much smaller group of foods that you'll be able to tolerate after getting a gastric band.

One of the questions I hear most often from weight-loss-surgery patients is, *Do I have to give up these things forever?* If you want to maintain the weight loss forever, the answer is yes. If the only reason you weren't eating foods that are high in fat, sugar, and calories early on after surgery is because they made you feel sick, then you'll find that you begin to tolerate these foods again about 2 years after surgery. But even though your body may be able to tolerate these foods again after a while, you need to make a long-term commitment to stay away from those concentrated calories if you want to lose weight and keep it off.

The other thing you have to give up to a large extent is the freedom you had before surgery to eat with abandon, because even if you're free of your excess weight, you still need to structure your life so that you can make healthy choices for yourself every day. If you're going out, for example, you should make a list of restaurants where you know you can get healthy foods, or you should prepare a little food in advance and bring it with you. If you skip a bunch of meals, you're going to be hungry and you'll end up eating too fast, which will make you uncomfortable. Remember that vending machines and food trucks have mostly bad food choices available, as do *all* the places we get fast food. In the long run, eating healthy is worth it; many people eventually find themselves wanting to eat more healthfully because being free of that extra weight feels so good. The health benefits you'll enjoy if you follow the rules your weight-loss surgeon lays out for you are enormous. But these benefits can vanish as quickly as they came if you continually put the wrong foods into your body. Bariatric surgeons don't expect perfection, but we expect you to give your very best effort, every day. Does that mean that you're looking ahead at a life of deprivation? Absolutely not!

We all know someone who can eat anything and not worry about gaining an ounce. If you're reading this book, chances are you're not one of those lucky people. I know I'm not one of them. But when you finally realize that your health depends largely on your postsurgery behavior—in many cases your *life* may depend on the choices you make—you will find the strength and resolve to make the positive effects of weight-loss surgery last on your own.

Food for Thought:
A Dietitian's Perspective

by Jennifer Arussi, MS, RDN

People who have had weight-loss surgery have to make so many changes in their lives, including making permanent adjustments to basic activity such as what and how they eat every day. Patients are often scared that they won't know what to do, that they won't eat right, that they won't be successful. Many are even sad about the prospect of eating healthfully and eating less; they worry about feeling deprived of the comfort they've taken from food for most of their lives. Seeking the advice of a registered dietitian can be, for some people, the key to getting a handle on the dietary changes that will ultimately contribute to their weight-loss success and improved overall health.

From a dietitian's point of view, one of the most exciting results of having weight-loss surgery for people with diabetes, aside from improved blood glucose levels, is the relief from feeling hungry all the time. What happens for a lot of people who have type 2 diabetes, especially when their diets are not balanced with healthy carbohydrates and proteins, is that their bodies initially make more insulin, and that insulin may make them hungrier. When these people have weight-loss surgery, not only are their bodies making less insulin, but the "hunger hormone" ghrelin is also under better control, resulting in reduced cravings for carbohydrates and relief from constant hunger. And that's a big thing.

Most of the people who come to see me don't have a good handle on their diabetes. They may have been educated about this disease at some level, but they just don't have all the tools to attain and maintain healthy blood glucose levels and a healthy body weight. Some of these people don't even know what their blood glucose levels should be. And it's rare for me to see patients who test *postprandial* blood glucose levels (where they test after each meal) rather than just testing their fasting blood glucose. If you check your postprandial blood glucose 2 hours after your first bite of a meal, that's the best way of monitoring how what you've eaten affects your blood glucose levels. Your blood glucose should read *below* 140 mg/dL 2 hours after each meal. You can use this target as a guide to help you determine what you can and cannot eat. For example, if you had 1 cup of pasta with 3 ounces of protein for dinner and your blood glucose was at 140 mg/dL 2 hours after the meal, it's probably okay to enjoy that same meal again another day. But if you overdid it one day and ended up eating 2 cups of pasta with 3 ounces of protein, and your blood glucose after that meal was 160 mg/dL, you know that you really need to watch your portion size the next time you eat pasta. Checking your postprandial blood glucose levels is one of the best ways to manage your diabetes, though not everyone with diabetes needs to test their blood glucose daily. Ask your health-care team if testing your blood glucose after meals is appropriate for your situation.

The people I meet with, whether they've already had weight-loss surgery or are considering it, have been on every diet in the world and, like most dieters, they have not been able to lose enough weight or sustain their weight loss. Some of them have been trying to lose weight since they were young children, unfortunately, and it's been their number one struggle in life. I find that so many of the people who have struggled with their weight feel that it is the *one thing* in their lives that they cannot overcome, despite their success in other areas of their lives. They've really tried multiple times in multiple ways to manage their weight, but

> **"So many of the people who have struggled with their weight feel that it is the *one thing* in their lives that they cannot overcome."**

without sustaining any substantial results. This is why weight-loss surgery is so appealing.

For those people who do opt for surgery, it is essential that they have some sort of plan in place for healthy eating after surgery. I think half the battle of weight-loss surgery is knowing that you actually went through with the surgery and that it can be helpful in setting your eating boundaries. But understanding ahead of time what those boundaries are—and making peace with them—is going to be critical for any patient's long-term success. There are so many things that you can't ever do again after you have weight-loss surgery, and for a lot of people these lifestyle changes need be understood and, if possible, practiced before the surgery.

So how do dietitians get patients to comply with these lifestyle changes? We take it on a case-by-case basis. If I have a patient whose issue was soda, for example—he or she just *loves* soda—I might initiate a conversation about what it is that's so special about soda to that person. Is it the carbonation? Is it the sweetness? Let's say it's the sweetness. I might then discuss with that person alternative ways to enhance the flavor of "allowed" beverages so he or she can enjoy sweetness without the need for carbonation.

While I like problem-solving with patients individually so we can talk about what their favorite beverages and foods are (their guilty pleasures), they need to know that adherence to post-op rules is still critical to their long-term success and that there are some non-negotiables when it comes to postsurgery lifestyle changes. (See Chapter 9 for a list of post-op rules.) They need to know what those non-negotiables are in advance, and they need to make peace with them. I remind patients to keep their eye on the prize. If they can do that, they can say, "Who cares that I'm not going to have alcohol for a year? This may be rough for me, but guess what? I'm going to have rapid weight loss. I'm going to be able to eat smaller portions of food and not feel deprived. I'm not going to feel hungry all the time. And I'm not going to feel upset with myself for not succeeding, because this time I'm going to finally start seeing progress!" There are so many big payoffs that they're going to get by adhering to the post-op rules, so they need to recognize that they're not *really* losing, but gaining!

There are many patients who do fine in their new postsurgery routine but eventually have to face the holiday season—which for many of us starts at Halloween and goes through Valentine's Day—with all its temptations that are so difficult to avoid. I recommend that you try to be as compliant as possible early on after surgery (0–6 months) to try to stretch out your honeymoon period. Later, when you're a year and a half or so out from surgery, if you want to occasionally have a bite of something sweet or find alternatives to sweets that you can manage and tolerate well, I think that is the key to lifelong happiness. I do believe you need to have *some* guilty pleasures now and then, because life needs to be exciting and, no doubt, food is pleasurable. I think part of the reason some people hesitate to have weight-loss surgery is because they think about the things they'd have to give up, and they worry that they're entering a life of deprivation. Personally, I think that mindset is so wrong. If you think about it like that, it seems so daunting. Try to think about all the good things you'll gain by having surgery. Once you're in it, you're *in it*, and most people don't regret it.

Having guilty pleasures is important, but you also need to *manage* those pleasures. I know many patients who have learned to manage their guilty pleasures and still maintain their weight loss. They no longer use food in the unhealthy way they used to because they have that parameter of their new stomach stopping them from eating copious amounts of high-fat, high-sugar foods. While most gastric bypass patients experience it less frequently as time goes on, some patients, even years after surgery, may experience some gastrointestinal distress or dumping syndrome. Eating properly after surgery is a lifelong commitment. You need to maintain an every-single-day, every-single-meal awareness, forever. And if you're going to put something in your mouth that doesn't belong there, you have to do it with awareness; you can't just start shoveling it in, because that's how weight is regained. I think that most people who have weight-loss surgery make that shift and become very conscientious about what they're putting in their mouth, and how they're eating. However, you always hear stories about individuals who ate too fast out of habit, or waited too long to eat and ended up with gastrointestinal distress or regurgitation. So the take-away here is to pay attention to those unfortunate bodily consequences and keep your head in the game. If you overeat or find yourself frequently indulging in foods you should be avoiding, take some time to regroup. Say to yourself, *I made a mistake here, and I can do better.*

Speaking of keeping your head in the game, I am a big proponent of food tracking. And while I have some patients who will disagree with me, I don't think that food tracking has to last forever. I think that, especially in the early phases following surgery, it's a good idea to track your food to make sure you're reaching your protein goal. (You should be getting in about 75–100 grams of protein per day.) Find a method of food tracking that works for you, whether it's a traditional pen-and-paper tracking system or electronic self-monitoring, so you can develop the keen awareness of what you're eating that is so important, especially early on. Later on, if you notice your old eating habits creeping back—if you're grazing or having a problem with excessive sweet consumption, for example—you may want to increase your accountability by re-engaging in self-monitoring practices. So I think food tracking is a good tool to help you increase your self-awareness and accountability. You can also always enlist the support of a health-care provider if you need that additional outside help staying on track.

Here are a few of my favorite tips for helping my patients achieve and enjoy well-deserved weight-loss success:

1. *Track your food.* As I already mentioned, keeping track of your food is one of the best ways to maintain accountability and make sure you're aware of your choices.

2. *Choose a protein shake.* Before you have weight-loss surgery, find some protein shakes that you actually enjoy. As discussed in Chapter 9, you'll need to eat a lot of protein after surgery, so protein shakes are going to be a staple in your life. Experiment with different blends and different flavors. Try adding a little fruit for some flavor variety, or some decaf coffee for a mocha shake. Find ways to like the shakes and make peace with them. I recommend doing this early, because if you wait until the day of surgery to figure out what protein shake you want to drink, it's going to be a longer, more difficult journey.

3. *Find a support system.* Enlist support from your family and friends and talk about how they can contribute to your success. For example,

let's say you meet a friend regularly at a favorite Mexican restaurant. Request that, instead of meeting at that particular restaurant, you go for coffee or a walk instead. And get yourself into some kind of support program (we can't stress this enough). Hopefully, the hospital or surgical center where you have your surgery is affiliated with a support group. Speak to other patients who came before you; they've been in your shoes. Ask them questions and learn from them. Try not to do everything on your own, because the truth is you've probably tried to lose weight on your own already and it hasn't worked out so well. So surrender and tell yourself that this time you're not going it alone.

4. *Enjoy your food.* Once you're through the early postsurgery period and you're starting to eat solid food again, find foods and recipes that are delicious and that you truly enjoy. Don't just find them, but actually *make* them! One thing that you need to remember about weight-loss surgery is that you're going to be eating such a small volume of food that what you're eating needs to give you maximum flavor and enjoyment. You're not going to be eating plain quinoa with steamed vegetables every night; that's not the goal here. The goal is to embrace the idea of eating healthy, but find a special flavoring to make those vegetables delicious or that quinoa palatable. You want to create maximum enjoyment from the minimal amount of food you'll be eating, so become a master chef in your own kitchen.

5. *Find ways to be active.* This is a lifelong *necessity*. Find your groove with physical activity. Sign up for 5K walks or runs, go to the gym, find a workout buddy, do exercise DVDs at your house, or take hikes…whatever works for you. Ask your friends and family what kind of activity they're doing so that you can partner with them, since it's easier to be active with a buddy than it is on your own. If you need to, hire a trainer to get you into the gym. Whatever way you do it, be active. That's the one variable that will help guarantee that you can sustain the weight loss that you achieve.

6. *Embrace meal planning.* A person who has recently had weight-loss surgery can't just walk out the door and expect to be able to navigate an entire day's worth of healthy eating. You have to anticipate what your day is going to look like and bring foods with you if need be. The moms out there will remember that, before you left the house when your children were little, you had to have the baby bag with all of the food and bottles and toys and diapers packed and ready to go. That's the same mindset you need to adopt now. Think about what you may need to bring before you leave the house so that you're not tempted to stop for fast food if you get hungry. Instead of grabbing unhealthy foods when you're on the go, you'll be prepared with a protein bar, an egg, some string cheese and some vegetables, or a piece of fruit. Planning is really the key.

    You can stretch your meal planning success by not only planning for each day, but trying to plan your entire week. The ability to plan meals that far in advance is a special skill possessed by only about 5–10% of the patients I work with. It takes a special kind of person to do that, but it's a good goal to work towards. Sit down with your significant other (or just yourself) and look at the week ahead. Make sure you have all of the groceries you need on hand and you know what you're going to prepare. You may even plan for a restaurant outing or two. Of course, plans can change at the last minute, but if you have appropriate food already in the house, it makes rolling with the punches a whole lot easier.

7. *Create a supportive food environment.* It's essential for you to cultivate a positive food environment for yourself, both at home and at work. Keep go-to foods on hand in the fridge, in cupboards, and even in desk drawers. Ditch the cookies. Remember: out of sight, out of mind. Plan to have a special shelf in the cupboard or fridge that is just yours, and fill it with healthy foods. Family and friends need to understand your difficulty managing chips, pretzels, nuts, etc. If they don't understand, set limits to make it easier on you. Remember, you deserve this!

8. *Engage online.* Use online groups and/or social media to exchange ideas and keep the food selection and preparation process exciting.

Websites and blogs dedicated to weight-loss surgery are often a great resource for postsurgery recipes. And there are several books available on the topic of eating after weight-loss surgery. Also, check out Pinterest, Twitter, and any other social media site that you find helpful and supportive (and fun).

There is so much great information out there for weight-loss-surgery patients; you just have to find resources that are appropriate for your particular situation, issues, likes, and dislikes, and make the recipe and ideas you find work for *you*.

—*Jennifer Arussi, MS, RDN, is a registered dietitian in private practice in Encino, CA. She specializes in weight-loss surgery and diabetes management.*

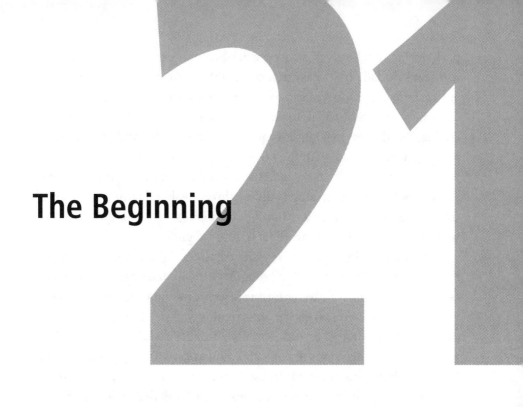

The Beginning

If you have read this book in its entirety, you've probably learned many things about diabetes and weight-loss surgery that you didn't know before. You may be thinking, *Thank goodness! I've finally made it to the end.* Well, sorry to disappoint you, but this isn't the end. In fact, it's just the beginning of your journey. Unless you're a glutton for punishment, I've got to believe that if you've made it all the way through this book, you are struggling with a significant weight problem (or you know someone who is).

When you decided to even consider the idea of weight-loss surgery, you had, no doubt, tried everything else you could think of to lose weight. You probably found a little success and a lot of frustration. But your health is at stake. Chances are you either already have diabetes or are headed that way. You may also be suffering from any combination of hypertension, shortness of breath, sleep apnea, bad knees, bad hips, or bad back—the works. *This is it,* you've said, *I want this fight to be over.*

But weight-loss surgery is not the end of the fight. It's only the beginning. It's the start of a very long journey which, ironically, may get even longer the more you progress, because you're taking steps to greatly improve and, no doubt, extend your life! You may think it's a walk in the park during that lovely postsurgery honeymoon period, when weight just seems to fall off. It's easy to lose weight at first, especially for the gastric bypass and sleeve gastrectomy patients who may experience the extremely unpleasant symptoms of dumping every time they taste a cookie. But that easy weight loss goes away, doesn't it? And after that, the willpower to continue with the postsurgery lifestyle has to come from within—from the very same place you accessed before surgery whenever you cut out carbs, or ate grapefruit for three meals a day, or microwaved frozen boxed meals from any number of sources, or drank diet shakes until your eyes crossed in an effort to lose weight.

So if you're lucky, and if we've done anything right in presenting this material to you, this will be the *beginning* for you, the beginning of your taking control—of your weight, your health, and your life. At this point, you should know how to get the information you need to make the decision about whether or not to pursue weight-loss surgery (one of the most important decisions of your life). You know what questions to ask. You know how important it is to listen to the answers and follow protocol. You have been reminded throughout this book that serious health problems arise from not having your diabetes and weight under control, and you know how essential it is to avoid these health problems if you possibly can.

As you've learned, even if you decide to have weight-loss surgery and succeed in putting your diabetes into remission, that doesn't represent the end of your weight-loss journey or struggle with diabetes. It is just the beginning of a transformation that takes a lifetime and involves completely changing one of the longest and most compelling relationships in your life—the one you've had with food. After surgery, food is no longer your buddy, your pal, your companion, or your comfort. That doesn't mean you'll no longer enjoy food; that is not the aim of weight-loss surgery at all. You just need to be aware of the choices you make because you don't want them to cost you your health or, ultimately, your life. Bariatric surgeons, and all health-care professionals, want their patients to live longer, happier, healthier, and more productive lives.

And weight-loss surgery is certainly not the end of the work. But it's the beginning of new eating habits, of an enjoyable, or at least bearable, fitness regime, and of a change in what motivates you every day. After surgery, it's the people and activities in life, not the food, that will motivate you. It's the beginning of feeling good, I mean *really* good, maybe for the first time in many, many years. It's the beginning of enjoying the success for which you are completely responsible. During this process you'll be learning new things, and you'll have the energy to pursue them. You'll also have the opportunity to share the knowledge you gain with others, especially those who may benefit from your experience. Weight-loss surgery allows many people to become the person their family deserves to have and be a participant rather than just a spectator watching life from the grandstand.

But if you want an ending, okay. Let's make today the end of a downward spiral of frustration, failure, and deteriorating health. Let's make it the end of joints that hurt, of physical exams that leave your doctor shaking his head, and of feeling disappointed in the person looking back at you in the mirror.

So you see, weight-loss surgery is not the end of the problem, it's the beginning of the *solution*.

Here's to your health!

Dr. Scott Cunneen

References

American Diabetes Association. Standards of medical care in
  diabetes—2016. *Diabetes Care* 2016;39(Suppl. 1):S1–112

Kassirer JP, Angell M. Losing weight—an ill-fated New Year's resolution.
  N Engl J Med 1998;338:52–54

Pories WJ, Swanson MS, MacDonald KG, et al. Who would have thought
  it? An operation proves to be the most effective therapy for adult-
  onset diabetes mellitus. *Ann Surg* 1995;222:339–352

Rubino F, Nathan DM, Eckel RH, et al. Metabolic surgery in the
  treatment algorithm for type 2 diabetes: a joint statement by
  international diabetes organizations. *Diabetes Care* 2016;39:861–877

Sjöström L, Lindroos AK, Peltonen M, et al. Lifestyle, diabetes, and
  cardiovascular risk factors 10 years after bariatric surgery. *N Engl
  J Med* 2004;351:2683–2693